Help for Hea
Other Books by L

Overcoming Back and Neck Pain

"The treatments recommended are practical, well described, and well illustrated...An invaluable resource."

—JOHN LABIAK, MD,
orthopaedist and spinal surgeon

"A very practical approach to the key things patients really need to know. I recommend it to all sufferers from spine problems...I appreciate Lisa's treatment of every person as someone who has not only a body and mind, but a spirit as well."

—KENT KEYSER, MS, PT, OCS, COMT,
ATC, FFCFMT, FAAOMPT
practicing and teaching physical therapist

Overcoming Overeating

"A practical, sustainable, and results-oriented approach that will guide you to permanent mind change...*Overcoming Overeating* provides both the why and the how toward becoming the new, healthy you."

—J. RON EAKER, MD
physician and author of
Fat-Proof Your Family

"A comprehensive remedy for weight loss. Lisa rightly views weight problems as having their origin in not just physical, but also mental, emotional, and spiritual arenas...An invaluable resource to the countless people struggling in this area of their life."

—DAVID HAWKINS, PhD
psychologist and author of
When Pleasing Others Is Hurting You

Get Healthy...for Heaven's Sake

"If you are looking to implement a healthier lifestyle, you will want to get a copy of this book...it isn't daunting like many books in this genre and it isn't restricting, but full of choices you can make to improve your lifestyle over time."

—BOOKSBARGAINSANDPREVIEWS.COM

"This book is a great resource, as it's not a bulky read. Instead, it's less than 200 pages and is full of information that can produce change in one's health, if applied!"

—THISMOMSDELIGHT.COM

Overcoming Headaches and Migraines

"A gift to headache sufferers and those in the health professions who are committed to helping them."

—HOWARD MAKOFSKY, PT, DHSc, OCS
head pain expert

"Lisa Morrone's extensive preparation, research, and years of experience are reflected in the safe and clinically proven techniques she recommends. A must-read for primary and specialty providers...and of course, anyone who suffers from headaches."

—WILLIAM ROBERT SPENCER, MD, FAAP
ear, nose, and throat specialist

Diabetes

"An easy-to-read, user-friendly guidebook for controlling or conquering the diabetes dilemma."

—READERVIEWS.COM

"This book...takes you on a journey through diabetes and then gives you a light at the end of the tunnel, teaching how to prevent type 2 diabetes and how to reverse the pre-diabetic state and metabolic syndrome. Should be read by everyone interested in living a full and healthy life."

—MARIANO CASTRO-MAGANA, MD
director, pediatric endocrinology and metabolism,
Winthrop Hospital, Mineola, New York

SLEEP
WELL
AGAIN

SLEEP WELL AGAIN

LISA MORRONE, P.T.

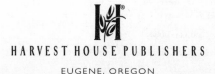

HARVEST HOUSE PUBLISHERS

EUGENE, OREGON

Cover by Koechel Peterson & Associates, Inc., Minneapolis, Minnesota

Cover photo © iStockphoto / Thinkstock

Back-cover author photo © Noelle D'Arrigo

Illustrations by Rose C. Miller

Lisa Morrone is published in association with William K. Jensen Literary Agency, 119 Bampton Court, Eugene, Oregon 97404.

Readers are advised to consult with their physician or other professional practitioner before implementing any suggestions that follow. This book is not intended to take the place of sound professional advice, medical or otherwise. Neither the author nor the publisher assumes any liability for possible adverse consequences as a result of the information contained herein.

SLEEP WELL AGAIN
Copyright © 2012 by Lisa Morrone, P.T.
Published by Harvest House Publishers
Eugene, Oregon 97402
www.harvesthousepublishers.com

Library of Congress Cataloging-in-Publication Data
 Morrone, Lisa, 1967-
 Sleep well again / Lisa Morrone.
  p. cm.
 Includes bibliographical references.
 ISBN 978-0-7369-2703-1 (pbk.)
 ISBN 978-0-7369-4256-0 (eBook)
 1. Sleep disorders—Popular works. I. Title.
 RC547.M675 2012
 616.8'498—dc23

2011022643

Printed in the United States of America

12 13 14 15 16 17 18 19 20 / BP-SK / 10 9 8 7 6 5 4 3 2 1

*"Come to me, all you who are weary…and I will give you rest…
learn from me…and you will find rest…"*

*Jesus' words from the Gospel of Matthew reveal to us that rest is first
off a gift and yet, at the same time, it is something we must pursue.
This book is written and dedicated to you—the tired, the weary, the
frustrated. May you find the healing, restful sleep that you long for.*

Acknowledgments

When my literary agent, Bill Jensen, first brought up the idea for a book on insomnia, admittedly I yawned. How interesting could I make the topic of sleep? *Well, even if it turns out to be a really boring read,* I jested, *it would still bring about the desired result, right?* Once I was knee-deep in my research, I found it was one of the most fascinating and needful books I could write. So, thank you, Bill. You're zzzz best!

From there I needed a sleep guide—and I found one in the very generous sleep expert Dr. Lee Shangold. Thank you for investing your time so that I could more clearly comprehend the complexities of sleep's architecture.

Thank you to those who have shared their sleep apnea testimonies within this book. You have allowed my readers a window into your own personal struggle with this potentially life-threatening disorder. I trust your life-changing outcomes will convince those with undiagnosed or untreated sleep apnea to not live another day without seeking a remedy.

For all the prayers of support that my Restoring Your Temple team has sent up as incense before the Throne, I once again thank you for your faithfulness. God continues His mighty work through us all.

To my husband, Peter—this is the sixth book in five years that you have read, chapter by chapter, and honestly critiqued. Thank you for pushing me to be the best writer and communicator I can be.

Finally to my editor, Paul Gossard, and my literary family at Harvest House Publishers—thank you for your attention to detail, every step of the way. I have been blessed and stretched for having joined you in this journey!

Contents

Foreword

by Lee Shangold, MD

Lisa Morrone has an uncanny ability to take a vast and complex field and break it down into easily understood components. I read Lisa's *Sleep Well Again* on a business flight from New York to San Francisco and found so much practical and useful information that I incorporated some of her explanations in a talk I was giving the next day on sleep apnea at a national meeting.

I am surely biased, but I believe that sleep is an important, timely, and fascinating topic. We spend one-third of our lives sleeping. When we sleep well, we don't think about it. When we don't sleep well, it is sometimes all we think about. From Hippocrates in 400 BC to William Shakespeare in the early 1600s to Charles Dickens in his 1836 novel, *The Pickwick Papers*, sleep and sleep disorders have been well described prior to any real understanding of these phenomena.

In its present form, the field of sleep medicine has been practiced for only the last 40 years. But what a 40 years it's been! The advances in diagnosis and treatment options for sleep disorders, over this short time period, have been nothing short of remarkable.

As is now known, sleep disorders can increase our risk of immune system dysfunction, high blood pressure, diabetes, heart attacks, strokes, and motor vehicle accidents. Poor sleep can lead to drowsiness, decreased ability to concentrate, memory impairment, decreased physical performance, hallucinations, mood swings and, in younger people, poor growth.

Since many of my sleep patients have more than one disorder, it is very common to focus on one diagnosis and then be somewhat disappointed when the adequate treatment of that one diagnosis does not lead to complete resolution of symptoms. However, Lisa's book is a comprehensive guide to the most common sleep problems—and if read in its entirety, will allow you to understand the vast majority of issues you might face.

Further, Lisa's writing is easy to understand and even easier to put into action. It gives practical suggestions about good sleep hygiene. It covers the entire spectrum of sleep disorders that can lead to poor sleep including insomnia, sleep apnea, restless legs syndrome, chronic pain, and others. I will recommend this book to my patients and keep a copy of it in my waiting room. After reading this book, I'll bet that you will "Sleep Well Again."

Lee Shangold, MD
Board-certified specialist in otolaryngology and sleep medicine
Clinical instructor, Montefiore Medical Center/Albert Einstein
College of Medicine

Chapter 1

So Tired of Being Tired

The March of the Weary Soldier

can feel my alarm clock staring at me, beckoning me to open my eyelids and take a peek. I resist and try to fall back to sleep. But as I lie there, the temptation to know grows stronger. I finally give in and lift one lid long enough to focus on the numbers. 3:13 a.m. Ugh. I try to force myself to get back to sleep. But instead I begin doing the math… adding up the number of hours I've already slept, and then the number of hours between now and the time my alarm is set to ring. "If I don't fall back to sleep soon, my day will be doomed from the start…"

And now, the very thought of dragging myself through the next day with burning eyes at half-mast has pushed my anxiety button. So I spend the next two hours tossing and turning, fretting more and more with each passing hour. An hour later, after I finally fall back to sleep, the inevitable happens—my alarm clock rings! Let the weary day begin…

Most everyone experiences a bad night's sleep from time to time. One sleepless night every few weeks, while troublesome, is not usually of great concern. It's when these nights of broken sleep begin to pile up, becoming more the norm rather than the exception—then there's a problem. *Sleep deprivation*, which by definition is getting *less than 7 to 8 hours of sleep per night*, has set in. Relentless nights of

insufficient sleep steal your energy, your focus, and your creativity—
not to mention your joy.

And poor sleep is stealing your health as well. It is well documented that the lack of sufficient sleep will significantly raise your
risk of injury both at home and at the workplace, increase the odds
of your being in a fatal traffic accident, and adversely affect your longevity. To put it starkly, sleep deprivation leads to life deprivation.

"Styles" of Sleep Problems

You may have trouble falling asleep. Night after night *sleep initiation* eludes you for one reason or another. Some of you can't get the
thoughts swirling around your mind to retire when you're ready to.
For others, physical discomfort is the reason you can't get comfortable enough to drift off to sleep. Or possibly you bring to bed a plate
piled high with stressful emotions,which you begin to chew on as
soon as you turn off the lights. Many of you, without realizing it,
have picked up some bad bedtime habits that are sabotaging your
sleep efforts. If trouble initiating sleep is your nighttime issue, be
encouraged. This problem is often easily repaired.

Some of you are thinking, *I can fall asleep—my problem is I
can't stay asleep!* For you and others like you, nighttime waking is
an unwanted guest in your bedroom—like someone leaning over
you and shaking your shoulder until you regain consciousness. (For
those of you who are parents of little ones, this may be literal rather
than figurative.) Some people find they wake prematurely from
stressful dreams or anxious minds, while others are wakened by nagging physical pain—headaches, neckaches, or backaches, shoulder
or hip pain, or a burning sensation in their midsection. For those of
you who are in your second half of life, many of you may wake to the
"sound" of your bladder alarm going off, compelling you to make an
unwanted trip to the bathroom. Still others of you haven't a clue as
to why you are suddenly awake—you just are. This book will offer
many suggestions that will work together to enable you to *stay* asleep.

A third "style" of sleep deprivation takes the form of *early-morning wakefulness*. You fall asleep quickly and sleep soundly, but unfortunately, you just can't seem to make it last long enough to be considered a full night's sleep (7 to 8 hours). This is often the case when mental and emotional stressors are so prominent that as soon as the opportunity for wakefulness presents itself, the brain shakes off its slumber and your mind is off and running. (I know this one well.) The early-morning wake-up call is also associated with aging. But it doesn't have to come along with getting older. You'll find many easy-to-apply tips throughout this book that can lead to a fuller night's slumber and a brighter daybreak.

For those of you who sleep with a partner, your sleeping problem may have nothing to do with you. It's *your partner's nighttime noises or motions* that are interrupting your peaceful night's sleep. If you share your bed with a snorer, then you know the drill—try to fall asleep quickly before they do. When your partner tosses and turns or jerks and flails, your bedroom takes on a "rock and roll" atmosphere that denies rest for the weary. And for those parents who share your bed with your children: Everything from nursing to little feet kicking to nighttime potty runs is likely to be disrupting your sleep.

If your rest regularly gets shortchanged, then I imagine you are desperate for a seamless night's sleep. In fact, you're likely in search of many of them. You're done with taking mandatory naps or nodding off here and there during the day. You're tired of dragging your deflated self through the day—each and every day—so tired, in fact, that you've bought this book (knowing you'll have the time to read it during your many wakeful hours). You're hoping it can shed some light on how you can get a better night's sleep and wake up refreshed instead of ready for bed again!

While this book is not a cure-all, it is a cure-*most*. The major factors that may be preventing you from sleeping well will be investigated and addressed, chapter by chapter—*bladder problems, physical pain, sleep apnea, restless legs syndrome, overactive brain, and even your own pre-bedtime behavior.* Furthermore, in chapter 10, we'll discuss the most popular sleeping aids available on the market today. This way you'll have enough information to allow you, along with your physician, to make an educated decision about whether or not to begin using these herbal or medicinal remedies. Finally I will wrap up with an appendix aimed at getting the teenagers in your life a better night's sleep, so they can set the stage for a lifetime of being well-rested.

But before we jump into the main course of this book, let's begin with an appetizer plate of sleep terms that will aid you in diagnosing, labeling, and treating your own sleep misbehavior.

Insomnia

When I hear the term *insomnia,* cartoon images from my childhood come to mind. I picture a weary character dressed in a long-sleeved nightshirt, slumped in a parlor chair in the dead of night. Beside him on a table stands a lit, burnt-down candle. His eyes have been devilishly propped open with toothpicks to prevent him from ever getting some sleep. Poor guy. Lack of necessary sleep is certainly agonizing. For those of you who have lived through nights that seem as tormenting as this, it's probably not surprising to you that sleep deprivation is used as a form of torture the world over.

Since the term *dyssomnia* (see sidebar below) is not in most people's vocabulary, those who have trouble sleeping typically say they are suffering from *insomnia.* The word *insomnia* literally means "no sleep"—which can actually be misleading. People who suffer from insomnia often report that they don't get any sleep. However, what is nearer to the truth of the matter is that they are not getting *enough* restful sleep. There are three qualifications that must be present in order for you to be diagnosed as having insomnia:

1. You experience poor sleep—either trouble falling or staying asleep, or poor-quality sleep.

2. Your poor sleep has a deleterious effect on you (mentally or physically) during the day.

3. This sleep problem occurs even though you have the opportunity to sleep and a favorable environment in which to do so.

There are different ways the medical field has chosen to classify insomnia. The most common classifications are based on its cause (*primary* or *secondary*) and duration (*transient, short-term,* or *chronic*). From the definitions below you can begin to qualify and quantify your particular sleep problem using standard terms.

DYSSOMNIA

This fancy word, when translated literally, means "bad sleep." And while everyone has an occasion of bad sleep, this term is more accurately used when describing ongoing sleep problems. As lonely as you feel sitting up all by yourself when everyone else appears to be asleep, you are most certainly not alone. Dyssomnia affects one out of every three adults each year to one degree or another, yet only 5 percent seek medical help.[1]

As we began to discuss above, the reasons behind dyssomnia are numerous. It can result from physical or chemical factors, or neurological or emotional issues—or a combination of these. Regardless of the cause, when you suffer from dyssomnia, consistently getting less than six hours of shut-eye per night, the quality and quantity of your life are significantly diminished.[2]

Primary Insomnia

When sleeplessness is not found to be caused by an underlying medical, psychiatric, or environmental factor, it is labeled *primary insomnia.* Sleeplessness *is* the problem; it's not the result of another problem. While some primary insomniacs have suffered with it since childhood, others have passed through a time of major or long-lasting stress that has altered their sleeping ability. Even after the situation has been resolved, long-term sleep disturbances continue to plague them.

Having endured this, many of these have developed a stress response whenever they approach the time of sleep. In addition to worry (*Will I be able to sleep tonight?*), other poor habits may have found their way into the life of the primary insomniac, such as regular nap-taking and going to bed extra early.[3] Both of these habits, while they seem to make the best of a bad situation, actually work against restoring a normal sleep routine.

Secondary Insomnia

In the case of *secondary insomnia* there are medical, emotional, or neurological reasons, or a combination of them, why one's normal sleep state has become disrupted. Sleep disruption is the symptom of another co-existing health problem. Below is a list of some of the major culprits fueling secondary insomnia (most of which we will be addressing in this book):

- headaches
- back pain
- neck pain
- other joint aches and pains, such as knee and shoulder
- heartburn (acid reflux)
- bladder conditions
- waking to breathe (sleep apnea)
- restless legs syndrome
- emotional upset, such as depression, anxiety, post-traumatic stress disorder

- major medical issues, such as stroke, overactive thyroid (Grave's disease), asthma, congestive heart failure, Alzheimer's, or Parkinson's disease
- menopause, hot flashes
- side effects of some prescription medications
- caffeine
- nicotine
- alcohol
- illicit drugs

Half of these causes for sleeplessness can be handled quickly, and better sleep can be restored to you as soon as tonight. Others will require a commitment to the appropriate medical or psychological intervention I recommend. But it is worth every effort that you make. You can regain the sleep you need to live a long and productive life by being proactive and addressing your sleep problem head-on.

Transient Insomnia

When your sleep is altered for just a few days in a row, you are experiencing *transient insomnia*. A work deadline or project overload can land me in this category a number of times throughout the year. While living with transient insomnia, my days become something to be tolerated and my nights something to be dreaded. You probably know exactly what I'm talking about.

Short-Term Insomnia

When sleep-altered days lengthen to two or three weeks, then you've advanced into the realm of *short-term insomnia*. Late-term pregnancy seems to inevitably do this to women. Between the aches and pains, the kicking baby (who never chooses to sleep when you

do), and the pressure on your bladder, welcome to months of interrupted sleep! A training ground, I always mused, for the sleep-
challenged months to follow.

Chronic Insomnia

When you battle with trouble falling asleep, staying asleep, or
getting a restful night's sleep that has lasted beyond one month,
your condition earns the distinction of *chronic insomnia*. You may
be experiencing months of sleep disruption while going through a
rough patch with your rebellious teen or if, sadly, you are facing a
divorce. Maybe your world has been altered by a job layoff or a life-
changing health diagnosis or physical ailment. In all these cases and
more, it is reasonable to experience dramatic changes in your sleep
behavior. For me, I've lived through months on end of interrupted
sleep due to back and leg pain. When my physical pain finally set-
tled down enough for me to sleep through the night, it took a while
to retrain myself to approach bedtime with a peaceful and welcom-
ing attitude, instead of worry and dread.

Whether you suffer with transient, short-term, or chronic insomnia, the cure may be right at your very fingertips. In the book you're
holding you'll find dozens of truly effective methods of alleviating
secondary insomnias…and even some of the troubling components
of primary insomnia. What remains is to determine what your specific sleep-disturbing issue is, or if you, in fact, have more than one
thing working against you.

Once you make that discovery, you can begin reclaiming those
lost hours of rest one step at a time. But as is the case with automo-
tive mechanics, it is vital that you understand the mechanisms of
sleep before we can begin diagnostics and repairs. Are you ready to
get started? Let's meet in the "body shop" in the next chapter.

Chapter 2

Eight Hours You Don't Want to Miss

The Amazing Architecture of Sleep

Most people think of dawn as the start of a new day. Not me. From the time I was a young child I have been influenced to consider the *evening* as the beginning of a new day. My father was responsible for my having this altered viewpoint. He was raised in an Orthodox Jewish home. Though he later converted to Christianity, he thought it important to teach me about the celebrations and observances of the various Jewish holidays and about how he had been taught to observe the weekly Sabbath. Each of these special days, without exception, began at sundown on the calendar day it was scheduled for, and then concluded at sundown either the following day, or whenever the festival days were set to end. So in my father's home, all cooking, cleaning, and other work-related tasks were to be completed on Friday before sundown in order to honor the Sabbath day of rest, which ran from Friday evening to Saturday evening...one complete day.

The other thing that had me convinced was Genesis (the first book of the Bible), where I found the account of God creating the first day. The earth was without illumination until the famous words of God were spoken: "Let there be light." In Genesis 1:5 it reads, "God called the light 'day' and the darkness he called 'night.' And there was evening and there was morning—the first day." Did you catch the order? Evening, *then* morning equaled the first day.

As I researched "all things sleep" for this book, the more and more it became obvious that indeed, the outcome of a day begins with what has occurred the night before. If we do not properly prepare ourselves for a good night's sleep (chapter 4), and if we neglect to investigate and seek resolve for the various health issues that work against our nighttime rest (chapters 5-9), then the next day will most assuredly begin with a significant handicap—physical, mental, and emotional weariness from sleep deprivation.

Sleep Needs Better PR

Even though few would argue that a good night's sleep makes for a good day, many adults still view sleep as a necessary evil—an interruption in the productivity of their day. We use phrases like "I guess I have to go to bed now" or "I should get some sleep." We've come by this attitude honestly. As children many of us fought naptime because it interrupted our playtime. We begged our parents to stay up "just a half hour later" so we could watch another sitcom. And if our innate childhood avoidance of sleep wasn't strong enough, some of our parents even used sleep as a punishment: "That's it! You're going to bed an hour earlier tonight!" As teenagers and college students, most of us stayed up as late as we could, shunning the very thought of napping—except, of course, for those homework-induced naps.

If you've coupled this negative attitude toward sleep with a limited knowledge of the benefits of sleep, is it any wonder you don't place a high value on your bedtime? Add to that the overloaded schedule you may be struggling to maintain, and voilà—you have joined the ranks of the sleep-deprived. Or maybe you really, really want to sleep. You know you need it in order to thrive and survive, but for one reason or another, a good night's sleep has eluded you.

According to the National Institutes of Health, there are 70 million people in the U.S. just like you—chronically underslept. In a 2009 study funded by the National Sleep Foundation, titled "2009 Sleep Poll America," researcher Michael V. Vitiello compiled some stunning findings:

- 46 percent of those who responded said their sleep needs aren't being met

- 35 percent said they sleep *less than six hours a night*

- 27 percent of those surveyed said they had disturbed sleep in the past month due to financial worries

Sadly, the same study discovered that the number of people who reported getting eight hours of sleep on a regular basis had decreased, from 38 percent in 2001 to 28 percent in 2009.[1] That's a 10 percent decline in well-slept individuals in less than a decade. If we keep staying up like this, we are going to become a nation of zombies!

THE NEW "U.S. PLEDGE OF ALLEGIANCE"

*I pledge allegiance to the Busyness of Life in the United States of
America,
and to the Rat Race for which it stands,
One Nation,
Underslept, Irritable,
with Fatigue and Weariness for all.*

Contrary to what many may think, sleep is not a state of nothingness—a mere loss of consciousness. It has, in fact, been architected with great refinement and purpose. Because of this, you simply cannot continue to upset the balance between wake and sleep in your life without reaping some serious consequences (chapter 3).

The rest of this chapter explores the amazing architecture of sleep. Once you realize all the incredible things that are happening in your

body while you're asleep, I'm positive you won't want to shortchange
yourself of even a half an hour of it.

Sleep's Control Knobs

We humans need sleep. If we attempt to hold it off, it will eventually come anyway. We cannot fight the natural inclinations imbedded into our design. Awake, asleep, awake, asleep; it is the cycle of
life. When it comes to sleep regulation or oversight, the body is
equipped with four mechanisms that influence its sleep and wake
states. As a result of their combined activity we are told when to fall
asleep and when to wake up. As long as these systems are allowed
to run without interference you and I will experience a timely shift
from nocturnal sleep to daytime awakening and back to nighttime
sleep once more.

To grasp this process more fully let's take a brief look at how each
of these control mechanisms work. Also we will make note of what
can happen to throw each of these four mechanisms off kilter and
wreak havoc with our sleep cycles.

Falling Asleep—The Homeostatic Process

The balance between wakefulness and times of slumber is man-
aged by the *homeostatic process*. Basically, the longer you are awake,
the sleepier you will get, until the time comes when you feel so far
out of balance (teetering toward sheer exhaustion) that you simply
must sleep.[2] As with a pendulum on a grandfather clock, you can
only swing in one direction for so long before you must return.

The awake → asleep component of this process is very much
influenced by the buildup of a waste product of living called *adenosine*. The more adenosine you build up, the sleepier you will get. Caffeine can add to your wakefulness because it works directly against
the lullaby effect of adenosine. Because caffeine runs interference,
blocking adenosine molecules from attaching to your brain's adenosine receptors your brain reacts as if a troubling emergency were

at hand. It responds by ordering your adrenal glands to release a dose of adrenaline—the fight-or-flight hormone—which gives your body an extra jolt of "awake." The perfect one-two wake-up punch!

We busy humans can also alter the sensitivity of this homeostatic process by repeatedly pushing our daytimes further into the nights. By burning the midnight oil year after year, we can become desensitized to our own sleepy feelings. I'd bet we're unique in the animal kingdom when it comes to this habit-formed sleep disturbance.

Staying Asleep—The Arousal Threshold

Once you have fallen asleep the *arousal threshold* mechanism kicks in. It acts as a buffer of sorts by keeping your brain insulated from wakeful disturbances (for example, noise, pain, and so on), allowing you to remain asleep. (Picture your brain with noise-cancelling headphones on.) As with any buffering system, there is a threshold, or point beyond which the barrier becomes insufficient. If your sleeping environment, either external (noise, heat, light) or internal (pain, anxiety), becomes too "noisy," your arousal threshold will be passed and your sleep cannot continue. But as long as the intensity of sleep-disturbing irritants remains under its set threshold, your zzz's will continue.

If you have had the joy of raising an infant or the privilege of caring for a sickly family member, then you know that your nighttime arousal threshold can be significantly lowered. When I brought my first baby home from the hospital, I had a storybook vision in mind for how we would spend our nights together. That first evening we placed my sleeping daughter in her eyelet lace–draped bassinet and rolled her up next to my side of the bed. Then my husband and I climbed into our bed to settle in for the night—or so we thought.

While my hubby dozed soundly that night, I was immediately awakened by every sigh, grunt, or whine that Casey made. After five hours of startle reaction on my part, I finally leapt from my bed in a state of utter exhaustion and rolled the baby-filled bassinet down the hall to the nursery. My arousal threshold had reached an all-time low. As a result, it took little to set off my mommy-alert button. It would be years before my threshold would rise to near normal levels. I say "near normal" because I don't believe that women ever fully recover from the heightened alert mode that comes from raising young children.

The Timing of Sleep—The Circadian Rhythm

Circadian rhythms are physical, mental, and behavioral changes that follow a roughly 24-hour cycle. They respond primarily to light and darkness in your environment. While not synonymous with your biological clock, your circadian rhythm has a significant influence on your sleep patterns. Your body's master clock is located at the base of your brain—more specifically in the *suprachiasmatic nucleus* (SCN) of the *hypothalamus* portion of your brain, which is seated just behind and between your eyes. (I added this bit of "GPS information" for those of you who have an understanding of anatomy and the desire to know.)

Interestingly though, it is the SCN that controls the production of *melatonin*, another hormone that makes you sleepy. Since the SCN is located just above the optic nerves (which relay information from the eyes to the brain), it readily receives information about incoming light. When there is less light—like at night—the SCN tells the brain to make more melatonin so you will get drowsy.[3]

Jet lag can thoroughly disrupt your circadian rhythm—especially when you're traveling from west to east. For every time zone you pass through, figure it will take you about 12 to 24 hours to reset your circadian rhythm. For example, if you cross six time zones, you can count on needing three to six days to feel normal again. (Provided you felt normal to begin with.) Living in places like Alaska, where there are extended periods of much daylight or much darkness, and enduring time changes caused by the switch to or from daylight savings time, can also influence your circadian rhythm.

Sleep's Arch Rival—Autonomic Nervous System Activation

Your *autonomic nervous system*, or ANS, is your body's hard wiring, if you will. Its functions enable you to adapt to changes in your environment. Known particularly for its fight-or-flight functions, the ANS controls hormone production, breathing and heart rates, body temperature, and wakefulness, among other things. When the ANS is activated, sleep will not occur.

Activation can occur because of external or internal influences. Examples of external activation are the ingestion of stimulants such as caffeine, or the presence of loud noise. Internal activation can result from fear, worry, physical pain, or anger. So whether it becomes activated before you fall asleep (you've just had an argument with a family member), or is turned on after you've been sleeping (you heard a startling noise), the result is the same—you're wide awake.

The Structural Design of Your Sleep Cycle

The introduction of the *electroencephalogram* (EEG) in 1929 led to a vast new awareness of the intricacy of the biological activity known simply as sleep. This recording device offered scientists a noninvasive way to measure the electrical activity of the brain. Through the use of surface electrodes, the electrical impulses sent back and forth between the brain's nerve cells could be documented and studied. It was from these studies performed on sleeping subjects that we came to understand the specialized architecture of sleep.

Through careful study of these EEG recordings, scientists discovered something surprising. While sleep seems to be uniform to the outside observer, the brain's internal electrical activity (or brain waves) was not consistent throughout the night. In fact, they found that sleep consisted of unique patterns of brain-wave activity that differed from one another in their amplitude (intensity or height) and frequency (rate of occurrence or speed). As if following a choreographer's lead, each pattern of electrical brain activity, after persisting for a set period of time, would then transition into another brain-wave pattern, or *stage*.

In 1968, researchers Kales and Rechtschaffen set forth a standardized way (revised in 2007 by the American Academy of Sleep Medicine) to describe the various stages of brain activity that had been discovered. They were *wakefulness*, *non-REM sleep* (subdivided into stages *N1, N2,* and *N3*), and *REM sleep*. Non-REM describes the state in which there is no *rapid eye movement*. In other words, during these stages, your eyeballs are resting from their activity of looking about. The REM sleep stage is characterized by the presence of rapid eye movement—both eyes are fully engaged, darting back and forth in a synchronized way.

In addition to the insight on brain waves and sleep stages, EEG recordings demonstrated that once the brain's activity had transitioned through each of these unique stages, the process would began all over again—revealing that the cyclical nature of sleep was inherent to its design. Typically it will take a person *approximately 90 minutes* to complete all of the stages of sleep (though more accurately the cycles can range anywhere from 80 to 110 minutes).[4] If you manage to sleep restfully for a seven- to eight-hour period you should expect to experience about five of these sleep cycles.

Below, I'll begin by defining the unique characteristics of each stage of sleep. Then we'll go on to the important biological processes that have been discovered to take place at predictable times within this cycle, all while you and I are asleep. It's simply amazing!

N1—Fragmented Sleep

During the night, you will spend a total of 5 to 10 percent of your time in N1 sleep. When you initially begin your sleep voyage, it can take up to a half an hour before you enter into this phase for the first time, which is quite normal. Slowly you drift away from the land of consciousness and toward the land of "nighty-night." Sometimes you can even feel yourself being pulled back and forth between awake and asleep as if you are caught in the ocean's tide. That is why this phase is described as *fragmented sleep*—because you are partly awake and partly asleep. During this brief stage you may experience *hypnic jerks,* in which you have a sudden flailing of a limb or startle reaction from a sudden sensation of falling.

During this transitional phase your eyes move very slowly under their lids, your body's muscles begin to relax, and your brain's electrical activity begins to slow down as well. N1 sleep is characterized by the presence of *alpha waves* (short, rapid waves—see diagram 2.1). During this stage you are easily roused by a change in your environment—a twitch of your limb, a raised voice, a pet

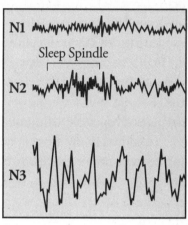

DIAGRAM 2.1

jumping on the bed. This brief time of transition from wakefulness to sleep lasts about *five minutes*, and then you enter N2.

N2—Light Sleep

This is the point in the sleep cycle where you've completely left the conscious world and have entered into a steady "asleep mode." Lasting an average of *55 to 60 minutes*, and taking up a total of 45 to 50 percent of your night's sleep, N2 is the longest phase of the entire sleep cycle. Aptly referred to as *light sleep*, N2 is similar to N1 sleep in that you can be easily woken from it—by a loud snore (yours or your partner's), someone suddenly switching on the lights, your partner flipping over in bed, your child calling your name, and so on.

EEG recordings confirm this phase of sleep by its characteristically unique brain-wave activity—*theta waves*, which are taller and slower than the alpha waves of N1. (See diagram 2.1 above.)

In addition, the brain-wave activity of N2 sleep is abruptly and irregularly interrupted by two other electrical phenomena. The first, *sleep spindles*, is recorded as bursts of rapid, rhythmical brain-wave activity imbedded among the slower theta waves. Research has revealed that sleep-spindle activity is related to an increase in recall performance and thus may very well reflect memory consolidation.[5] The second phenomenon, known as *K-complexes*, is characterized by a sudden increase in wave amplitude (height, or intensity). Studies have yet to determine exactly what the complexes are responsible for, but there are two emerging theories gaining acceptance. First, it is believed that K-complexes assist the body in remaining asleep by ignoring sleep disturbances. The second thought is that they, along with the sleep spindles, aid in memory consolidation. Stay tuned, though—the mystery may be solved before this book even comes to print.

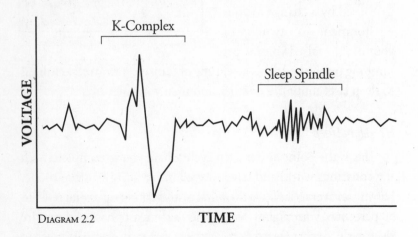

DIAGRAM 2.2   **TIME**

During N2, or light sleep, the body also undergoes some significant physical changes. Overall your skeletal muscle tone continues to drop, eye movement progressively lessens, your body's temperature lowers, and your heart rate begins to slow, all in preparation for the next stage—deep sleep.

N 3—Deep Sleep

As your brain-wave pattern changes for the next phase of the non-REM portion of the cycle, you will enter into *N3 sleep*, also known as *deep sleep*. As its name implies, it is very difficult to rouse someone during this stage. If you've ever been awakened abruptly during this stage, you probably felt terribly groggy and disoriented. It can take quite a bit of time to shake off the fog of deep sleep and begin feeling truly alert again.

N3 sleep is the shortest of the stages, accounting for just 3 to 20 percent of the 90-minute sleep cycle (somewhere between *3 and 18 minutes*). The older a person gets, the less time they spend in N3 sleep. Teenagers tend to spend closer to 20 percent of their sleep time here, while the elderly will spend a mere 3 percent.

During N3 sleep, the body is characterized by breathing that is deep and rhythmical, very low muscle tone, and a cessation of all eye movement. The theta brain waves of N2 sleep are replaced by larger amplitude (tall), *delta waves*. (Again, see diagram 2.1.) And if you are prone to sleep talk or sleepwalk, this is the time in the cycle that such *parasomnia* behaviors will likely appear.

THE BRAIN WAVE OF PAIN[6]

People who suffer with chronic pain caused by fibromyalgia, arthritis, disc disease, or the like know that just because they happen to be asleep, it doesn't mean their pain has taken a rest. When the brain waves of these pain sufferers are studied, an intriguing anomaly consistently surfaces. The brain of someone in pain produces alpha waves (normal to the N1 stage) during the N2 and N3 phases also—when there should be only theta and delta waves present.

The terms *alpha intrusion* or *alpha-delta sleep* have been coined to describe this predictable phenomenon. Since alpha waves are somewhat "wakeful" waves, it is hypothesized that although a chronic-pain sufferer does enter into N2 and N3 sleep, these phases lose much of their effectiveness due to the more wakeful intruders, and therefore the person awakes in the morning without feeling refreshed.

REM–Dream Sleep

As you and I enter into this final portion of our sleep cycle, our physical bodies and our brains' electrical activity once again switch gears, and they usher us into what's more commonly known as *dream sleep*. REM sleep is uniquely characterized by *rapid eye movement*—which is quite like how our eyes move about when we are awake and alert.

REM sleep accounts for 17 to 28 percent of our sleep cycle. And even though our dreams can sometimes seem as if they last the entire night, the time spent in REM sleep is usually only *5 to 15 minutes* per cycle. That said, the first sleep cycles of each night have been shown to contain relatively shorter REM periods and longer periods of N3, deep sleep. As the night progresses, REM sleep periods increase somewhat in length while time spent in deep sleep decreases. By morning, people spend nearly all their sleep time in stages N1, N2, and REM.[7]

In addition to bringing the incredible and often bizarre world of dreams, this last sleep stage also brings with it some specific alterations in the workings of our body. Our breathing changes from rhythmical and deep to shallow, rapid, and irregular. Our heart rate increases, our blood pressure rises, and males develop penile erections. And as this stage's name indicates, our eyes jerk rapidly in various directions as if we were watching our dreams play out on a movie theater screen before us—which might be somewhat accurate. And to ensure that we don't act out those dreams, as part of the design architecture of sleep, all the muscles in our bodies become temporarily paralyzed—with the exception of our heart, our diaphragm, and our eye muscles. Now isn't that incredible?

Sleep's Recipe for Restoration, Rejuvenation, and Readiness

Once it became common knowledge that the brain's electrical activity varied throughout the sleep cycle, an even greater dimension of the study of sleep was sparked. It was theorized that as the brain's electrical activity varied, so too the body must be experiencing unique biological functions or purposes associated with each stage. Researchers were right to follow their instincts, and you'll see below that what scientists have discovered is truly fantastic.

N1—The Prep Work for Sleep

Not much to mention here in the way of biological productivity. Though to give this stage its proper recognition—without actually *falling* to sleep, you and I would never get to *be* asleep. And then we'd miss partaking of all of the benefits of the further stages of sleep. So thank you, N1.

N2 and N3—The Pit Crew

Ever watch a long motorcar race, such as the Indy 500? At points within the excitement, each car will suddenly exit the racecourse and come to a screeching stop in its pit. During this brief intermission the pit crew descends upon the car and quickly tightens loose wheel bolts, tops off engine fluids, adds fuel, puts air in the tires (or swaps them out altogether), and then—*zoom*—the car and driver are back in the race!

This is how I picture all the biological fixes and fueling that happen during N2 and N3 sleep. We race through life at top speed, but when our body is on the verge of malfunctioning (signaled by weariness), we fall asleep (make a pit stop). When we veer off into N2 and N3 sleep a myriad of reparative and restorative processes begin to take place simultaneously.

All day and night the human body and brain send messages back and forth by way of electrical impulses. These impulses travel from nerve cell (neuron) to nerve cell until they reach their intended location (a neighboring area of the brain, your big toe, pancreas, or left eyelid). The heavy usage results in daily wear and tear on this critical system. If it were left unattended we would quickly find our nervous system malfunctioning.

Throughout the stages of light and deep sleep your body's electricians are called into work. It's at this midpoint within the sleep cycle that your body's nerves are systematically repaired and tested to assure perfect function for the day ahead. Nerves that are not given the required recovery time will begin to malfunction. Increased sensitivity to pain, neurologic tremors, spasticity, or rigidity all may be the result.

Beyond this, what science has discovered is truly fascinating. (I am sure they have just begun to scratch the surface.) First of all, during sleep our musculoskeletal system is fortified. Bones are rebuilt and strengthened, and muscle fibers increase in girth in order to meet the challenges that have been placed on them the day before. Without adequate restorative sleep, you could suffer from broken-down bones and frayed muscle fibers—namely arthritis (bone and joint wear and tear) and myositis (muscle inflammation and spasms). Fibromyalgia (a painful muscle disorder) has long been linked to chronic dyssomnia.

During N3, the deep-sleep phase, critical components of your chemical health are also being manufactured and distributed. Hormones such as insulin and growth hormone are produced by the pancreas and the brain respectively. Insulin maintains proper blood-sugar levels, and growth hormones, as you'll learn in the next chapter, prevent aging, among other crucial tasks.

Furthermore, neurotransmitters ("postal workers" for all those electrical messages sent along your nerves) such as *serotonin* (5-HT) are replenished and topped off. When the neurotransmitters of the brain are in short supply, all sorts of havoc occur—not the least of which are depression and anxiety. The pharmaceutical industry is supplying an alarming amount of serotonin precursor 5-HTP or serotonin re-uptake inhibitors (drugs which block existing serotonin from being reabsorbed and therefore, unavailable for use). Wonder if the fact that most Americans are underslept has anything to do with that?

REM Sleep—The Finishing Touches

Everyone would like to know exactly why it is we dream. While there are many theories, no one really knows for sure. The one thing we do know about this fourth stage of sleep is that it is absolutely necessary for our survival. A study performed on rats led to this discovery. While rats normally live for two to three years, those deprived of REM sleep survive only about five weeks on average! Much is still unknown about REM sleep, but what we do know is quite compelling.[8]

The one thing I find most fascinating has to do with my earlier mention of the fact that while we dream our arm and leg muscles are paralyzed. So get this—the reason our muscles need to be unplugged, beyond protecting us from acting out our dreams, is so our bodies can repair and sequentially test each muscle connection. Now isn't that a fabulous design trait?

Interestingly, it has been discovered that during this brief time we are dreaming our brains are also busy sorting through, consolidating, and filing away new memories made during the previous day. While we no longer need to remember where we parked our car in the grocery-store parking lot, we do need to recall our new ATM personal identification number or the name of our child's new teacher.

Finally, if you ever wished you could improve your golf swing or work on a newly acquired dance step while you sleep…you can. Brain studies have shown that while you are in this dream stage, your brain is reviewing newly learned physical movements. It runs through the nerve firing sequence over and over, so that you can wake up and perform better than you did the day before. In fact, people who were taught a skill and then deprived of non-REM sleep could recall what they had learned after they woke up, while people deprived of REM sleep could not.[9] Now if that isn't fascinating, I don't know what is!

The Wonders of Sleep at a Glance

Here is a handy sleep-benefits chart to remind you of the crucial importance of getting seven to eight hours of sleep each night. Use it to educate a family member or share it with a friend. Maybe then you can hold each other accountable to sleep well so you can live well.

BIOLOGICAL PROCESS	N 2	N 3	REM
Nerves repaired and tested	X	X	
Bones rebuilt	X	X	
Muscles fortified	X	X	
Hormones replenished	X	X	
Neurotransmitters produced	X	X	
Muscle connections repaired and tested			X
Memories consolidated			X
"Virtual practice" of skilled body movements			X

Let's be clear on a final point: If you lose a quarter of your sleep time to wakefulness, you will gain only 75 percent of the built-in benefits of sleep. That means 25 percent less hormones and neurotransmitters produced, 25 percent less time to rebuild nerves, bones, and muscle, 25 percent less time for your mind to prepare itself to assist you in your daily life.

In the following chapter we'll examine, in detail, the health consequences of chronic sleep deprivation. Once you are armed with the facts from this chapter and the next, I believe you will be thoroughly motivated to tune up or even overhaul your sleep behavior—whatever it takes.

Chapter 3

No Snooze? You Lose

The High Costs of Sleep Deprivation

Growing up I was convinced I was missing a gene—the "staying up late" gene. In college while all my peers were up past midnight having fun or studying, I was unable to join them. I was bushed and in bed by 11 p.m.—no matter what. Even a looming anatomy exam couldn't keep my eyelids open. I cannot tell a lie—I've spent most of my adult life envious of those who seem to function perfectly well on less sleep and more coffee.

My first boss did nothing to lessen my envy. John was a model of productivity. He could work a full-time job, head a busy family, volunteer in his church and community, and still have time to pursue advanced degrees and develop professional seminars. People would often ask in amazement how he could possibly accomplish so much, all at the same time. He would lean back his head, smile broadly, and chuckle that he "only needed" four hours of sleep each night.

John's easy response always made the frustration I had over my own "inadequacy" that much greater. My life seemed to be moving at a snail's pace next to his accomplishments, and I was at least ten years his junior. Saddled with my pathetic need-to-sleep condition, I resigned myself to the fact that I would never accomplish as much as he could—not with all the sleeping I had to do.

Well, ten years after I had begun working for John he was diagnosed with lymphoma, seemingly out of nowhere. No problem. Everyone knew he was a strong, get-it-done sort of guy. Surely this cancer would be no match for him. Three months later he was gone—much to everyone's shock and disbelief, including my own—at the age of 43. How could this have happened? He had seemed so healthy...

Fast-forward another ten years. While researching the topic of sleep for my last book, *Get Healthy for Heaven's Sake*, I came across this eye-opening statement from Dr. William Dement, the cofounder of Stanford University's Sleep Center:

> There is plenty of compelling evidence that sleep is the most important predictor of how long you'll live.

Could it be that those lost hours of sleep had deducted years from John's life? While that premise can never be proved, scientific research certainly stacks the odds in favor of the lost sleep → lost health → lost years of life scenario. One such piece of evidence came from a British study published in 2007, which found that life spans were diminished for people who slept less than 7 hours per night.[1]

From that time forward I began to view my sleep handicap as a gift, rather than a curse to be endured. By viewing sleep as a health-improving, life-extending part of your day, I believe you too can gain the motivation you need to strive toward gifting yourself with a full night's sleep, seven days a week, as far as it depends on you.

It's Time to Get out of Debt

We've already established that getting less than seven hours sleep per day is defined by the experts as sleep deprivation. Think of it this way: If sleep were a currency measured in minutes and hours, loss of adequate sleep over time would leave you overdrawn, unable to pay the bills of life in full. The lifestyle habit of lost sleep results in serious debt, *sleep debt*.

Further, *your sleep debt is cumulative*. Week by week, month after month, and with each passing year, your body is keeping an account. Because you began life with a solid balance in your account, it can take decades before your account begins to read "red." However, you can only run in the red for so long before the bill collector comes knocking—in the form of sickness, disability, or even death.

Beyond Tired—The Health Consequences of Poor Sleep

Many people are convinced that the worst part of a diminished night's sleep is the tiredness of the next day. That is the least of their worries. Because such a vast array of physical, chemical, and electrical housekeeping duties and next-day preparations occur while we sleep, getting just 75 percent of your required sleep is like driving out of the pit stop during the Indy 500 before your fourth tire has been secured! Your sleep behavior will have cut short your recovery from the previous day, leaving you at higher risk for a crash—physically, mentally, or emotionally. Let's break down what could be causing the breakdown.

A Foggy Mind

As we get older, many of us complain of brain fog. The mental clarity of our past seems to be a thing of the past. In response, some people will begin to take mind-stimulating substances and herbal remedies such as ginkgo biloba or ginseng. Yet how many of us have ever thought about getting a bit more shut-eye to sharpen our brains?

It sounds simplistic, but research has proven that something fabulous happens to alter our brains while we sleep. In addition to all the body-restoring activities we saw in the previous chapter, during non-REM and REM sleep (N2 through REM), the brain is busy growing new backup cells. This is imperative, because as we age we do begin to lose brain cells, beginning as early as age 30! In addition, sleep allows the brain to construct alternate nerve routes (communication pathways) to connect our existing brain cells. (Picture it this way: Adequate sleep allows for the production of new brain "cars" and "roadways," so our brain's traffic—thoughts and calculations—can continue without so much as a slowdown.)

The amazing BDNF. In order for all this construction to take place, however, there must be a specific chemical present in the brain. Dr. John Ratey, author and brain expert, refers to this crucial chemical as "Miracle-Gro for the brain." Its proper name is *brain-derived neurotrophic factor,* or BDNF. And wouldn't you know it? BDNF is produced while we sleep. With sufficient supplies of this brain fertilizer present, your body can bolster its brain cell count. Consistently achieving a full night's sleep enables you to build up and train a strong brain reserve (much like the Army Reserve). So the next time an old communication pathway in your brain fails to complete its mission, you can rely on your backup brain reserve to come to the rescue.

Not only does sleep debt make you brain-cell deficient, but it also affects the function of the cells you do have. Case in point: Brain scans have shown sleep deprivation to have a deleterious effect on the frontal cortex of your brain. (This is the part of your brain that is seated right behind your forehead.) Its job responsibilities include being your decision-maker and high-level thinker among other functions.[2]

Inadequate sleep has been documented to result in dulled and inefficient thinking. I know I feel this sort of "brain molasses" whenever my sleep has been interrupted. Still another study found that people were less effective in making executive decisions (making up their minds and following through) after missing *just one night* of sleep.[3] So if you find that you struggle with indecision or dulled and inefficient thinking, according to this study, sleep could very possibly become your cure.

Less than seven hours sleep per night can also affect your ability to think through problems. Which of us hasn't gone off to bed facing some sort of dilemma? We've put off making a final judgment until we've had time to "sleep on it." Why is that? Well, while you are sound asleep, your brain has been found to use that downtime to analyze, problem-solve, and even learn![4] I find it quite remarkable that we can go to sleep and wake up smarter. So if you're looking to improve your ability to properly analyze information, getting some extra sleep tonight is the way to do it.

Making memories. Here's yet another mental problem we tend to chalk up to getting older—a poor memory. *Where did I leave my car keys...eyeglasses...the pen I was using?* Perhaps you've attended a church service or a workplace seminar and you've struggled the next day to recall what was taught. Well, you've been created with an "app" for that—the *hippocampus* portion of your brain.

The hippocampus functions as your brain's memory maker. It is a paired structure sitting behind your right and left temple (you know the place you tap when you are trying to remember something?). In addition to forming new memories, the brain power we gain while sleeping helps us to access old memories as well. Research has confirmed the connection between sleep and memory by identifying that sleep-deprived people actually have lower activity in the temporal lobes of their brains—the location of these marvelous hippocampus structures.[5] If memory, mental clarity, and a sharp intellect are important to you, you can preserve these traits with a full night's sleep.

A Sickly Body

The immune system is an amazing creation. It was designed to always be on high alert, ready at all times to hunt down "body invaders" and annihilate them. But if your immune system becomes weakened, it can be inadequately prepared to wage war against those ill-intentioned intruders. Repetitive sicknesses and the onset of many diseases may very well be the result of a malnourished immune system, one that has been starved by poor sleep. One study I came across clearly demonstrated that all it took to measurably weaken your immune system was just one five-hour night of sleep. [6] This is probably why so many college kids return home sick after their midterms and finals are over.

When things really go awry in our immune system, it begins to assault the very body it was designed to protect. Autoimmune diseases such as multiple sclerosis (neurological deterioration), lupus (an inflammatory disease affecting joints, skin, kidneys, blood cells, heart, and lungs), and Hashimoto's disease (insufficient thyroid hormone production) are examples of an immune system wreaking havoc on its host body. I am not claiming that gaining more sleep will *reverse* autoimmune diseases, but if we live life with a sleep-deprived immune system, we may be at greater risk for an "immune system coup." So if you are frustrated by frequent illnesses or fighting a life-altering disease, then do your immune system a favor—address your sleep problem.

An Expanded Waistline

Who would have thought that a lack of sleep could be bad for your body weight? Yet study after study shows a direct correlation between what is termed *short sleep* and obesity. [7] Likely you've had the experience of being completely ravenous the day after a particularly bad night. You eat everything in sight and then hunt for more. People who've had this happen to them surmise they must be looking for extra energy in the form of food calories. Not necessarily. Something even more ominous is occurring. While there are many factors that lead to hunger, the basic desire for food is largely controlled by two appetite-regulating hormones produced in the brain. These hormones are manufactured in perfect balance when you sleep 7 to 8 hours per night.

When you spend less time in deep sleep (N3), the production of these two hormones gets thrown out of balance. The first such hormone, *leptin*, tells your brain when you are full. It is an appetite *suppressor*. The second and competing hormone, *grehlin*, is an appetite *stimulant*, letting you know, loud and clear, that you are hungry. With less than seven hours of sleep your brain will produce excess grehlin, the appetite stimulant, and not enough leptin, the appetite suppressant. This flip-flop in production of hunger-controlling hormones leads many people to pack on excess pounds that wouldn't materialize if they had only slept better.

Altered Emotions

Many people live their lives in silent mental anguish. Chronic emotional pain can lead to clinical depression, which has been found to affect 20 million Americans annually.[8] Many men and women who live under the weight of depression have been diagnosed by their physicians or psychiatrists as having a chemical imbalance. The chemical in question is the neurotransmitter serotonin (introduced in the last chapter—a.k.a. 5-HT).

Scientific researchers have come to believe that depression is basically the result of either an insufficient production of serotonin or the decreased ability to utilize what is available. Because of this, clinical depression has often been treated (and somewhat effectively) with prescription medications that alter the amount or utilization of this neurotransmitter within the brain. The most widely prescribed group of medicines in use today are the *selective serotonin reuptake inhibitors* (SSRIs), which act to keep more serotonin floating around or in play to be used. SSRI's include such commonly recognized brand-name drugs as Prozac, Zoloft, Paxil, and Lexapro.

Now, the crucial point: Serotonin production and time spent sleeping go hand in hand. As I mentioned in the previous chapter, brain neurotransmitters are produced during the phases of light and deep sleep (N2 and N3). If you cheat yourself out of just one 90-minute sleep cycle, you will have effectively depleted your stores of serotonin by 20 percent. Is a full night's sleep enough to get you off your medication? Maybe not, but it could help to diminish the dose you need to be effective—and any time you can take less medication, your liver will be that much happier.*

Being Accident-Prone

Growing up, I had a younger brother our family had labeled "accident-prone"—though we used the Italian word *stunata,* which means "head in the clouds." It seemed he was always getting injured, usually because he wasn't aware of his surroundings. We used to believe it had something to do with his propensity to daydream. Well, all that daydreaming allowed him to develop into a highly skilled painter. And the bumps, cuts, and bruises are now (for the most part) a thing of the past.

That is not the sort of "accident-prone" I am referring to here. Though the results of klutziness or distractedness are sometimes entertaining, sleep-induced accidents are no laughing matter. You are often in grave danger when you are underslept. Numerous studies have found that sleep deprivation dulls our senses and slows our reaction time. In addition, sleep debt leads to poor judgment and decision-making, which only compounds the situation. In fact being awake for 24 hours straight has been found to have the same physical effect as having a blood-alcohol level of 0.10 percent—the equivalent of consuming six alcoholic drinks![9]

Nonetheless, only in the state of New Jersey is *D.W.D.,* or Driving While Drowsy, a punishable offense. Under their "Maggie's Law" (named after a 20-year-old killed by a sleeping driver), any driver who causes a fatality after being awake for 24 straight hours or more can be prosecuted for vehicular homicide.[10] I wish more states would follow suit—for the safety of everyone on the road. From 1999 through 2008 it was determined that *nearly 17 percent of fatal car crashes were the result of D.W.D.*, according to Peter Kissinger, the president and CEO of the AAA Foundation for Traffic

---

* Never attempt to adjust your medication dosage without the supervision of your doctor.

Safety.[11] More people have nodded off at the wheel for a moment or two than would likely admit it—but you know who you are. If you are so tired that you can't keep your eyes open while behind the wheel, you are taking a frightening risk.

Workplace, home, and public-location accidents caused by fatigue and sleep debt are further examples. These incidents can result in a broken ankle, a lost limb, or something much worse. Notorious and enormously costly workplace disasters in which sleep deprivation was involved are the wreck of the supertanker *Exxon Valdez*, the *Challenger* space shuttle explosion, and the nuclear reactor catastrophes at Chernobyl and Three Mile Island. One person's poor or nonexistent night's sleep can have a devastating effect on the world around him.

It may be that you have spent most of your adult life in a state of sleep deprivation. The day-to-day worn-out feeling seems quite normal to you. Momentary snoozing and brief catnaps may be an accepted part of your life. Well—they shouldn't be. A well-rested person should not begin to feel sleepy until bedtime nears. (No matter how boring your activity is.)

Give yourself a wake-up call by taking the quick quiz below. This way you'll discover whether your sleep debt–induced weariness should be cause for concern.

THE EPWORTH SLEEPINESS SCALE

In contrast to just feeling tired, how likely are you to doze off or fall asleep in the following situations? (Even if you have not done some of these things recently, try to work out how they would have affected you.) Use the following scale to choose the most appropriate number for each situation.[12]

0 = would never doze
1 = slight chance of dozing

2 = moderate chance of dozing

3 = high chance of dozing

Situation	Chance of dozing
Sitting and reading	
Watching TV	
Sitting inactive in a public place (for example, a theater)	
As a car passenger for an hour without a break	
Lying down to rest in the afternoon	
Sitting and talking to someone	
Sitting quietly after lunch without alcohol	
In a car, while stopping for a few minutes in traffic	
Total	

A total score of greater than 10 is a definite cause for concern, as it indicates significant excessive daytime sleepiness.

Accelerated Aging

Anti-aging products and procedures are big business in this country. The old notion of aging gracefully has failed to translate to the present generation. No sirree, we are promised much more on TV ads and in magazines—apply this cream, have this facial peel, a nip here and a tuck there…and you will look ten years younger. And men are also getting plastic surgery and the like at higher rates than ever before. The narrowing job market is what I believe to be one factor here.

What if you found out you have the best and least expensive anti-aging process at home, and it is found right there on top of your pillow? You're right, it's sleep—but I bet you could have guessed that answer by now.

Back in chapter 2 we saw that the brain produces growth hormone while you are in the two non-REM stages of sleep (N2 and

N3). While growth hormone functions to cause a child to grow to their full stature, it continues to have important growth functions even after we're full-grown. An adequate amount of growth hormone thickens your skin—making it firmer and suppler. No creams, ointments, chemical peels, or surgery required.

Growth hormone is also of critical importance because it allows us to maintain our bone and muscle mass. Bone loss for women (osteoporosis) can lead to pain, deformity, and fractures. Moreover, your strength (muscle mass) wanes with age. Strong bones and shapely muscles not only protect our bodies, but they enhance our looks as well. If you shortchange yourself of this true-to-its-name "beauty sleep" you will run low on growth hormone. Next time you meet someone who looks good for their age, ask them how much they sleep at night. My bet is they'll answer, "Seven or eight hours."

Sleep deprivation also accelerates aging in another way. It has been connected to increased risk of heart disease, heart and brain attacks (stroke), type 2 diabetes, and insulin resistance. All these may stem from another hormone you don't have time enough to make in adequate amounts—insulin.

Abbreviated Life

From rats to humans, research study after research study confirms that lost hours of sleep lead to lost years of life. You have a lot to sleep for! To review, sleep was designed to

- repair structural damage incurred throughout the day
- build brainpower
- bolster your physical strength
- recharge your immune system
- refuel your body's hormones, neurotransmitters, and other critical compounds

All of these factors work together to allow your body to function optimally. Just like the nighttime work crews on the highway, the construction gets underway when you turn out the lights.

I have come to believe that sleep is one of the six pillars of good health. (If you're curious about the other five, pick up my previous book, *Get Healthy, for Heaven's Sake*.) You need to sleep, and you need to sleep well. You need to sleep, and you need to sleep long enough. With sleep, make it your goal to "chase it down and capture it" so it can sufficiently do the job it was intended to.

So how do you do that? Follow me to the next chapter and we'll look at how you can get yourself ready for a good night's sleep.

Chapter 4

Getting Ready for a Good Night's Sleep

How to Be on Your Best Bedtime Behavior

Anyone who has played sports or who has given a speech would agree that proper preparation leading up to the game or event can really stack the odds in favor of a great performance. You may have never considered sleep something to be "performed," but in many ways the act of sleep can be very much affected by how you prepare for its arrival.

The vast majority of you reading this book suffer from secondary insomnia—insomnia caused by an underlying medical, psychological, or environmental factor (see chapter 1). Thus there is much that you can do, preparation-wise, to make sure that you are on your best bedtime behavior. There may be sleep-challenging internal factors going on inside your body, such as nighttime bathroom runs or back pain, which can successfully be put to bed. Perhaps you'll discover there are environmental sleep-saboteurs you've been living with, which have been fighting against your shut-eye. Or maybe you'll find that there are habits, behaviors, or routines you've incorporated into your life that are working against your best sleep intentions.

In this chapter we'll first identify your particular cause or causes of secondary insomnia. Following that are some terrifically practical fixes for you to put in place so you can give those sleep-deterrents a rest. Then in chapters 5 through 9 we will focus on a handful of secondary factors that I believe warrant a full chapter to address adequately—namely medical problems affecting the bladder, obstructive sleep apnea, restless legs syndrome, and an "overactive brain." So let's begin with some scene changes, shall we?

Setting the Stage for Satisfying Slumber

Environment, or physical surroundings, is so very important—when enjoying a meal in a restaurant, while watching a theatrical play, and when setting the stage for a peaceful, uninterrupted night of sleeping. Here are six staging components that every serious sleeper must have in place.

Cut the Lights

This shouldn't come as a surprise, but you were created to sleep best in a dark environment. In fact before the lightbulb was invented, people slept ten hours per night on average! Nowadays people attempt to fall off to sleep in front of the flickering light of their television, with the bold red alarm clock numbers beaming at them, and sometimes with their partner's reading light on. All this is no good.

A number of years ago I attended a continuing education course on the subject of sleep. Interestingly, the instructor told us that research had found women to be nine times more sensitive to light than men. No wonder I can't fall asleep quickly when my husband is still up reading…and when I "spring" my clock ahead for daylight savings time, I'm up at dawn. If you and I want to fall asleep quickly and stay asleep, we need mood lighting, which in this case is *no* lighting.

Light-dousing ideas:
- Turn off the TV.
- Install room-darkening window treatments.

- Use your cell-phone alarm or turn your clock face downward to decrease its brightness.

- Gift your partner with a small reading light or an illuminated glass page cover for bedtime reading—just bright enough for them, and dark enough for you.

Adjust the Temperature

Sleep experts agree that your bedroom temperature is best kept somewhere between 65 and 72 degrees F. Why is this important? In the second chapter we talked about how, during N2 (light sleep), the body's temperature must drop to help induce sleepiness. If you are overheated, your "sleep chase" will be more difficult. Similar sleep disturbance can happen if your bedroom is kept too cold. While your body will try its best to keep itself at a preferable sleeping temperature, it is incapable of regulating its own temperature during REM sleep. Therefore, you can be pulled back into the land of wakefulness during this stage *by becoming either too hot or too cold.*

Temperature regulating ideas:

- Buy an inexpensive thermometer to determine what the actual temperature is in your bedroom.

- In the winter, use a dual-control electric blanket when sleeping with a partner. This way you'll both feel comfortable.

- Use an air conditioner, ceiling fan, or supplemental heating unit to protect against extreme seasonal temperature swings in the bedroom.

Cue the Quiet

Is your bedroom a place of peace and quiet? Or if the sleep fairy were to magically appear, would she find your TV blaring, your iPod earphones in your ears, and full-throated conversations under way just before you roll over to sleep? There's just one thing to say: Hush the noise!

Noise-dampening ideas:

- Foam earplugs work wonders…especially if you sleep in a noisy city or with a log-sawing partner.
- Simply unplug from all sound-wave-producing items.
- Keep conversations to a low tone, and don't discuss any issue that may cause you to get upset and tempt you to raise your own voice. Save that for morning.

WHITE NOISE

For some, sleeping in a silent room just doesn't work. They need a sound to drown out all the other sounds. Enter white noise. *White noise* is produced by combining sound waves of all different frequencies together. The sound of an operating floor fan closely resembles white noise to the human ear.

Since white noise contains all frequencies, it can be used to mask other sounds—ones that would potentially disrupt your sleep. It does this by overwhelming your brain's ability to distinguish one frequency from among so many (like trying to hold a conversation at a wedding while the reception room is filled with 200 guests and an enthusiastic DJ).

Funny story—one of my brothers has slept with a blanket-covered box fan whirring since he was a teenager. When he came to visit me as a bachelor, his fan always came too. My husband and I used to remark that it would be difficult for him to find someone who would put up with all that noise—that is, until the day he met his wife-to-be and they discovered they both slept best when a fan was running. There really is someone for everyone, isn't there?

Put Out a Casting Call for New Bedding

When you have sleep problems, you don't want to add insult to injury by trying to get comfortable on an old lumpy mattress and a deflated pillow. Once your mattress has served you for a decade, it is time to seek a replacement. Patients ask me all the time which mattress is the best. The truth is, just like with shoes, bedding comfort depends upon your body structure and your sensitivities. I believe that mattresses that are firm, yet have a moldable topper of sorts (to fit into all your "nooks and crannies"), seem to work the best for comfort and support. As for pillows, I like to replace them every three years, but that will depend on their ability to meet the supportive criteria (see chapter 6 for details). Sheets and blankets (and even pajamas) that are cotton and breathable also help you to avoid overheating.

Clear the Stage

I have seen a lot of bedrooms in my days—those of children, teens, and adults—and therefore I can honestly say I have seen a great deal of clutter. I don't know how so much stuff makes it into the bedroom, but it does. Laundry to be folded, papers to be sorted, bills to be paid, mounting piles of once-read books, newspapers and magazines, last season's decorations that never made it into the attic—you name it, you'll find it in a cluttered bedroom. If you want your mind to drift peacefully off to sleep, it helps that the last waking scene you encounter is a peace-giving, calm, orderly environment.

Restoring-order ideas:

- Methodically remove all items from the bedroom that do not pertain to sleeping or dressing.
- Be diligent about tidying up your bedroom surroundings.

- Make your bed. It is a more calming "stage set" to
  climb into at night.

Animals and Children—Exit Stage Left

I am not anti-pet or anti-child. (Although ever since our family's English springer spaniel had to be put down at the ripe old age of 13, my kids have joked that I "hate" pets. Not true—I dislike the mess, the extra work, and the pet-sitter fees I had to pay for over a decade…but I digress.) Anyhow, I believe children and pets are a welcome addition to the home—just not to the bed. All that jumping on and off the bed, wiggling, changing positions, random kicking, and yelping…it's a wonder anyone sleeps. Good thing my husband was in agreement with me when it came to child-rearing: Under no circumstance did our kids sleep in our bed. If our son or daughter needed comforting, we went to their beds, not the other way around. Our bed was off-limits to little people, and to our springer spaniel.

Taking-back-your-bed ideas:

- Set a new rule about who is allowed in your bed.

- Place a see-through child gate across your toddler's bedroom so they can't escape from their room into yours—they will call out and you can come to them.

- Travel back to your older child's bed with him or her should they wake and need some TLC.

- Scoot out the dog, cat, pig, or whatever it is you have taking up room in your bed and close the door—bed space is premium, and any extra startling movements or sounds at night are not welcome!

- Crate any animal that can't manage to contain itself at night in a faraway part of the house.

WHEN TO SAY NO TO NAPS

If you regularly have difficulty falling asleep at night or staying asleep for seven or eight hours, I strongly suggest you bite the bullet and eliminate naps from your daily routine—no matter how tired you are. Adults need to sleep approximately one hour for every two hours of wakefulness. So if napping is your common practice, you are already attaining some of that sleep time during the daylight hours. This routine makes it unnecessary for your body to achieve a complete night's sleep. It is a bad cycle to get yourself stuck in.

For those who have an occasional night of poor sleep, a quick nap to pay back some of the last night's sleep debt is not a bad idea. But here are the parameters of such a nap:

1. Nap duration should be either 20 to 30 minutes (to avoid entering the deep-sleep phase) or 90 minutes (one complete sleep cycle).[1]

2. You should never nap (not even a five- or ten-minute catnap) after 3 p.m.

It's All a Matter of Timing

Sometimes we derail a good night's sleep simply because we have our timing all wrong. I am not talking about the time at which you go to bed and wake up (we'll save that for later in the chapter). What I mean by timing is more a matter of scheduling. Throughout the day you work, eat, exercise (some of you, anyway), take medications, and so on. However, if you do any of these at the wrong time, they can work against your sleep, leaving you tossing and turning on your bed. Below are what often prove to be the biggest sleep offenders when not scheduled appropriately.

Caffeine. We are a nation that lives on caffeine. Coffee shops are on every city corner and in every suburban strip and shopping mall. Caffeine is a chemical stimulant which heightens our alertness—so for an underslept people group (remember 74 percent of Americans don't get adequate sleep), you can see why this substance has such a hold on us.

The problem is that this stimulant has a very long half-life (the time it takes for half of it to be flushed from your body). The actual half-life of caffeine varies from person to person, but it is about six hours.[2] So for most people, if you have your last dose of caffeine before 3 p.m., you should be in the clear by bedtime. However, if you are extra sensitive, back up that time recommendation by an hour or two. Remember, caffeine is found in coffee (even decaf to a lesser degree), black (nonherbal) teas, all chocolate, many soft drinks, and even in some pain meds (Excedrin) and daytime cold medications.

Alcohol. Often people confuse the sedative effect of alcohol with the natural drowsiness caused by our brain's hormone melatonin or the neurotransmitter adenosine (both sleep agents). So they have a nightcap to unwind and get sleepy before bed. The problem is that alcohol, while it may help you to fall asleep, has been shown to disrupt the deep-sleep and dream-sleep cycles (N3 and REM). It is also a diuretic, which means it will fill your bladder quickly, and that also could wake you at midnight. That is a pretty high price to pay. Now the half-life of alcohol is shorter than that of caffeine,[3] so you can still enjoy a beer or a glass of wine with dinner. Your best bet is not to drink alcoholic beverages within three hours of bedtime.

Eating and drinking. Here is where timing is everything. Eating too late at night is a real sleep-killer. Indigestion, acid reflux, and the feeling of being bloated are not what you want when you are lying horizontally. Be sure to schedule your day so that you don't commit the "sin" of working through dinnertime. And if you are accustomed to having a glass of wine or a beer with dinner, an earlier eating time will allow for that.

If you are dealing with middle-of-the-night bathroom runs (those not directly related to bladder or prostate issues—see chapter 5), timing of fluid intake is critical. If you drink too close to bedtime, you may find you can't hold your urine until morning. On the other hand, if you stop drinking too early in the evening you will wake—as I sometimes do—completely parched. The mere act of reaching for my bedside water bottle is enough, on some nights, to fragment my sleep and keep me awake for half an hour. So with everyone's stomach and bladder tolerance at different levels, you need to stay aware and discover what your best time is to enjoy your final meal and down your last beverage.

Work. Back in the day, most people who were employed worked their official hours and no more. There were no mobile phones or laptop computers to extend the workday into your evening drive home—or right on into the night.

These days the line between work and home is blurry at best (especially for those of you who, like me, work primarily from home). True, there is always more that needs doing. But if you want to keep on living so you are around to continue your employment, begin to erect some time boundaries (for example, absolutely no working after 8 p.m.). If your mind is engaged right up until the time you slide the laptop off your bed and turn the light out, sleep will likely elude you. Or if you do drop off to sleep immediately (due to exhaustion or sleep debt), you will likely have disrupted sleep and stress-related dreams when you finally reach REM sleep.

Exercise. As a physical therapist, I love telling people to exercise. But here you are going to hear me say something uncommon—*don't exercise.* Let me qualify that—don't exercise *within 3 hours of your bedtime.* Exercise is wonderful in so many ways: It lowers blood pressure, reduces body mass, increases the production of "happy" brain chemicals (endorphins, serotonin, and so on), stimulates brain-cell production, and improves strength and flexibility. But it is a stimulant nonetheless. And as such it raises your body's core temperature for many hours, which will work against the N2 stage decrease in body temperature, which in turn induces deep sleep properly. As with most things…with exercise, timing is everything.

KICK YOUR SMOKING HABIT IN THE "BUTT"

Smoking holds no redeeming qualities. Nicotine is an addictive stimulant that can truly sabotage a healthy night's sleep. By now you know that stimulants of any kind (chemical, physical, or emotional) mix with sleep like water with oil. In addition, because of the highly addictive nature of nicotine, your brain will actually wake you in search of a refill in the wee hours of the night, whether or not you give it what it's pining for. So lay down those smokes and sleep through the night.

Sabotaging Your Own Sleep

Recently I noticed some black scuff marks on my wooden floors. I tried to wipe them off with a regular sponge, then a scrubbing sponge—but alas, those streaks remained. So I had a lightbulb moment. I reached for my Magic Eraser sponge and voilà—the streaks melted away. So I gleefully went around my entranceway and living and dining rooms removing those blemishes one-two-three.

The problem showed up when my sponge swipes dried. My floors' clear coat had been marred by the abrasive in that magic sponge, leaving unsightly dull areas throughout the house. My intention and desire was to clean my floors, not ruin their finish. But ignorance of how my Magic Eraser was working against me sabotaged my cleaning efforts.

So it is with your sleep. You want a good night of sleep, and you have the best of intentions to get a good night's sleep, but unbeknownst to you, bedroom behaviors are sabotaging your best efforts.

TV. Long ago and far away, families had one television set (with rabbit ears) in their living rooms, where people did most of their living. Today in our world of overabundance, we've literally littered our home with them. As a result, most Americans have televisions in their bedrooms.

This is a bad idea on many levels, unless you are disabled and basically bedridden. The bedroom is supposed to be the place that, when you enter it, your body is conditioned to become drowsy. However, when you get into bed and click on the TV, your mind associates bed with excitement, drama, comedy, reality…you name it—everything except sleep. So if you want a more soothing and effective transition from awake to asleep, haul that baby out and make your bedroom a less stimulating environment.

Computers and the Internet. Desks in the bedroom are a new feature. It seems that as more homes were designed with master bedroom suites, many of us moved the office into the sleep station. Laptops and iPads have now enabled even those with small bedrooms to climb into bed with the company of the whole World Wide Web. Folks, ditch the technology. You need to settle your brain down to neutral before attempting to drift off to sleep. Working, gaming, surfing the net—it can all work against peaceful slumber. It is difficult enough to flush the thoughts of the day from your brain without adding an extra pile of thought trivia on top of it right before you slip between your sheets.

Work. As we spoke of before, the boundaries around work time have taken a major hit in our generation. But that just means you need to be even more diligent to stand guard against bedroom intruders—and work is definitely one of them. Working late into the night while propped up against your bed pillows will fight against the soothing, sleep-inducing atmosphere of your bedroom. Paperwork, cerebral reading material, laptop spreadsheets…all must be left outside the door of your bedroom. They will be there in the morning, and you will have a sharper mind to handle your tasks if you are well-slept.

Finances. I don't know many people who can think about, much less talk about, their personal finances without their heart rate rising. Paying bills, transferring bank funds online, or trying to balance your checking account should be done way before bedtime.

If you need the input of your partner on financial matters, don't launch into a discussion minutes before you are to turn in. Instead, make a date to discuss it over dinner, or at least during daylight hours. And whatever you do, don't ask emotionally charged questions of your partner, such as "How come we're in overdraft?" or "How much did you spend shopping today?" The only thing that comes from that is two agitated people tossing from side to side under the covers.

Stimulating reading. I love to indulge in a little reading before I drift off to sleep. I usually try to get into bed a half an hour before lights-out so I can relax with a few pages of an interesting read. But here is where you need to know yourself. If you are prone to get involved in a suspenseful fiction book, one that you simply can't put down (like my husband often is), you may need to trade that book for something less engaging, like a magazine, a hobby guide, or a short-story compilation. Before-bed reading is good, as long as it doesn't keep you up too late or make your mind rev after you've put it down.

Finally, reserve your bedroom for only two things: sleep and sex! While sexual intimacy is indeed stimulating for most people, it has the added benefit of hormonally driven postrelaxation effect on the body—especially for men. It's a great way to de-stress, reconnect, and ultimately, to relax.

Keeping Your Sleep Appointment

Perhaps nothing is more disruptive to achieving a solid night of rest than having your home, work, or travel schedule significantly alter your bedtime and waking time. How do you deal with this issue?

Altered bedtimes. The majority of people find themselves living two different lives—one during the week and the other on weekends. As we saw in chapter 2, unless we mess with it, our biological clock and circadian rhythm remain constant Sunday through Saturday. So too should your sleep and wake times.

The problem many people face is that they try to make up for their workweek's sleep debt by sleeping in on the weekends. Or they disregard the whole sleep-debt thing and just stay out really late on Friday and Saturday nights and sleep in the following mornings. Well, can you imagine the internal confusion suffered by your hormonally driven biological clock? At what time should it release melatonin—10 p.m. or 12 a.m.? When should it rouse you—6:30 a.m. or 10 a.m.? Fluctuations are inevitable, but they should be kept to a minimum—say one hour in either direction. That way you do not send mixed messages to the "fall asleep" center of your brain.

Working shifts. Millions of Americans deal with shifts at work. If you regularly work the night shift, then you need to be diligent about setting the stage for sound sleep (room dark, earplugs in, regular bedtime, and so on).

But if your shift changes on a regular basis (as is the case for many police officers and medical personnel), then you are in a very difficult situation. In fact, if sleep deprivation is an issue that concerns you and your longevity is at stake, I would seriously recommend a new job search. Some people can handle the constant change in their sleep schedules, but if you are not one of them, you may find it necessary to leave your job in exchange for a better life.

Jet lag. Recreational travelers know they need to deal with the inevitable jet lag resulting from vacation pursuits. They may have the luxury of even adding a day to acclimate. But what if your job has you flying out at a moment's notice, or has you crunched for time on both ends of your trip? What then?

When you must cross over numerous time zones, there is where the sleeping problems arise. In fact experts say that for every time zone you cross, it will take approximately one day to adjust. (For example, a trip from California to New York crosses three time zones and therefore will take a person a full three days to adjust.) The worst jet lag occurs when you are flying west to east because you lose part of your day and the nighttime arrives too quickly, throwing off your circadian rhythm. If your trip is for only one to two days, don't try to influence your sleep cycle—just bite the bullet and go with the flow. You'll be back home and on schedule soon enough. But if your trip is longer than two days, here are some tips which may help to make the transition smoother:

- When traveling *west* → *east* the best strategy is to begin setting your daily sleeping and eating schedule backward by one hour each day for two to three days prior to your trip.[4]

- When traveling *east* → *west* the best strategy is to progressively stay up at night one hour later and wake one hour later for two to three days before you travel. Adjust your mealtimes according to your new time schedule.[5]

Secondly, once you arrive at your destination you must make sure to manage your new sleep setting to your advantage. That means the bedroom is dark when you try to sleep, you don't eat too late or too heavy, and you have a comfortable set of earplugs with you. When you are trying to sleep on the plane, a sleeping mask (eye visor) and noise-canceling headphones can be real sleep savers.

ROUTINE MATTERS

Just like children, who behave best when they know what to expect, the human body was created to function optimally when a consistent schedule is followed. If you learn to condition yourself to settle down before bedtime by following a routine, falling sleep won't have to be such a wrestling match. As an example, below you'll find my regular going-to-bed routine :

1. Turn house lights lower in the evening time

2. Wash face, floss and brush teeth, and remove contact lenses

3. Retire to the bedroom

4. Turn off overhead light, so only bedside reading lights remain

5. Dress in comfortable, season-appropriate cotton (breathable) pajamas

6. Get into bed half an hour before I want to go to sleep

7. Read a book, magazine, or something else that is nonstimulating

8. When my eyelids get droopy or when bedtime arrives, close reading material and turn out bedside light

9. Pray briefly with my husband

10. Kiss him good night

11. Commence snoozing…

Healthy Practices That Promote Sleep

To wrap up this chapter I wanted to share three tried-and-true sleep improvement practices that you can apply to your life beginning this very day. Each one holds the potential of making a world of difference in the quality and quantity of your sleep.

Regular exercise. We already spoke about exercise in terms of the timing of it. But truthfully, even beyond the benefits that exercise brings to your strength, flexibility, blood pressure, brain health, immune system, and sugar metabolism, consistent exercise helps you to sleep better. In fact, research has repeatedly shown that exercise provides three critical benefits: you fall asleep faster, attain a higher percentage of deep sleep, and awaken less often during the night.[6] All these sleep bonuses (as well as all the other benefits of exercise) can be yours by performing as little as 20 to 30 minutes of exercise three to five times a week.

An "agreeable" diet. By "agreeable" I mean that not only should you eat a well-balanced diet consisting of ample fruits and vegetables, lean proteins, high-fiber foods, and plenty of water, but you should also regulate when and how much you eat throughout the day. Changing your dinnertime by over an hour or going out late for a heavy dinner with friends or clients can really upset your sleeping routine—not to mention your stomach. If you have problems with heartburn or acid reflux, then you need to be especially vigilant. (See chapter 6 for a sleeping posture suggestion if nighttime indigestion or reflux is a troubling issue for you.)

SELF-SOOTHERS

Sometimes life has us so tightly wound that we simply can't settle down without some sort of "intervention." For some, *a soak in a warm tub* by candlelight or with some soft music each night may be just what the sleep doctor ordered. Close your eyes and lie back. As the warm water soothes your muscles, imagine the stressors of your day just melting away. When you drain the tub, allow the "melted problems" to drain away too—if even just for the night.

Other people find a new sense of calm when they spend some quiet time in *prayer or meditation*. Reflective time can often help you break free from a me-centered mind-set and enable you to gain better perspective on the day's events. Choose to dwell on the good of the day.

Even in the worst of days there is much to be thankful for, if we'd only redirect our focus.

Another way to soothe yourself to sleep is to use *relaxation techniques*. One such technique involves simple imagery. Close your eyes and picture a multihued sunset. As you breathe in, imagine you are filling your lungs with all the colors of that painted sky. Exhale slowly and completely, picturing the stressful events of your day being expelled from your body in the form of smog. Repeat 10 to 20 times until you feel more peaceful.

Yet another relaxation technique often used by performers is one in which you isometrically contract the muscles of different regions of your body, followed by the relaxation and release of those same muscles. Begin with your face, then your shoulders, then arms, hands, abdomen, legs, and finally ending at your toes. This sequential contract-then-relax technique can help to release the burden of tension you've absorbed into your body throughout the day.

When you were an infant you soothed yourself to sleep by sucking on your thumb, pacifier, or milk bottle...so consider these methods grownup-sized pacifiers to use when you want to "make nighty-night."

Some R & R...and the other "R." The majority of Americans live life with the "pedal to the metal." Our lightning-fast pace leaves us utterly exhausted. When we feel as if we are on the brink of an emotional and physical breakdown, we take a vacation—usually somewhere expensive and far away...so we can unwind. Then it's back to life lived at full-tilt once more. The problem is that we are conditioned to believe that R & R (rest and relaxation) can only be enjoyed when we take a vacation from work. Truth is, if we incorporate some rest and relaxation—and some recreation (the other "R")—into every day (or at least into our week), we will be better balanced and therefore more capable of making the transition from day to night.

After everything we have considered in this chapter, I now wish you "good night." I'll see you in the morning—bright-eyed and bushy-tailed, I hope. Sweet dreams of better days—and nights—to come!

Chapter 5

"Oh No, I've Gotta Go!"

Fixing Your Plumbing Problems

For nearly a decade my family, along with four or five other families, went camping each summer in the Delaware Water Gap in Eastern Pennsylvania. At the end of each day we would sit around the fire until we could no longer keep our eyes open. Before turning in, each of us would visit the campground's bathrooms and then head back to our tents—and sleep all night long.

As the years went on, some of the adults in our group began to enter their fifties. Our once still, pitch-dark campsite started to see some nighttime action. Beginning about two or three o'clock in the morning, tent zippers could be heard opening. Flashlight beams cut through the darkness, and gravel crunched underfoot as someone hurried off to the bathroom. The problem got so bad for one member of our group that she installed a port-a-potty inside her tent so she wouldn't risk running into a bear in the middle of the night. Ah, the joys of getting older…

Can you remember the last time you slept straight through the night without the obligatory trip or trips to the toilet? If you're in your fifth, sixth, or seventh decade of life, you may wonder if it is even possible to restore a full night's sleep.

For most of you, I believe it can be done without much ado. All it will take is a bit of knowledge and some lifestyle revision (and being a physical therapist, I have to throw in an exercise or two). Though a few of you may require some medical intervention, even then, I believe you'll find that you can eventually break free from night-time toileting.

Quite often people have developed late-afternoon habits and pre-bedtime behaviors that stack the odds in favor of the unwanted bathroom runs. We discussed these trouble spots in the last chapter, but here we will recap some of these with emphasis on those that fill your bladder and empty your "sleep account."

What You Drink

Certain beverages act as *diuretics* in the body—which means they increase the volume of urine produced. Alcoholic beverages such as wine, beer, and hard liquor; caffeinated brews including coffee, tea, and soda; and surprisingly even grapefruit juice will send your kidneys the message to pump up the volume. These drinks are best avoided if you are suffering from a nocturnal need-to-go.

MEDICATIONS CAN PUT YOU ON THE RUN TOO

There are a group of medications used specifically for their diuretic properties to combat high blood pressure and alleviate water retention (edema) from congestive heart failure and some forms of liver or kidney disease. Sometimes they are simply referred to as water pills. Here's a list of such commonly prescribed medications that might be causing nighttime waking:[1]

Brand name	Generic name
Aldactone	spironolactone
Bumex	bumetanide
Diuril	chlorothiazide
Esidrix or Hydrodiuril	hydrochlorothiazide

Hygroton	chlorthalidone
Lasix	furosemide
Lozol	indapamide
Midamor	amiloride

When You Drink

Timing, as mentioned in the previous chapter, is everything. Researchers have found that the *half-life* of caffeine is six hours, whereas the half-life of alcohol is three. (The half-life is the period of time in which half of the chemical component is cleared from your body.) That being the case, it is best to not drink caffeinated beverages closer than six hours from your bedtime. And when it comes to having a nightcap or a final glass of vino—do it at least three hours before the time you plan to turn in. As for grapefruit juice, your best bet is to save it for earlier in the day.

FYI: GRAPEFRUIT AND STATIN MEDICATIONS DON'T MIX

Statins are a group of medications used to treat high cholesterol. And while we are talking about grapefruit juice I wanted to make sure you are aware of an important drug interaction and precaution.

Grapefruit juice contains a substance that blocks your intestines from breaking down certain medications, including the statin group—Lipitor (atorvastatin), Mevacor (lovastatin), and Zocor (simvastatin). As a result, your circulating blood level of the active ingredient in these medicines is significantly increased, which can result in a dangerous muscle disorder or possible liver damage. So if you're on statins, the benefit of lowered cholesterol far outweighs the cost of saying goodbye to this citrus fruit.[2]

How Much You Drink

Deciding just how much you can drink without overloading your bladder's capacity is best discovered by trial and error. Begin this experiment by stopping liquid intake about an hour before bedtime. If you still wake up, back it up by another half hour. Continue to do this until you find what works best for you. (There should be no need to go beyond three hours.) Here's a tip, though. Avoid eating super-salty foods or snacks (the kinds that create thirst) from the early evening on. This way you're not driven to drink!

Nothing says, "Wake up!" more loudly than a bladder in need of relief. Yet this should be a nonissue for us while we are asleep. We humans were created to go into "hibernation mode" when we are sleeping. Our body temperature drops, we are able to fast for eight hours without hunger pangs, and our kidneys respond by reducing the amount of water they pull from our blood, decreasing the overall volume of urine produced. It's therefore quite normal for a sleeping adult to be able to make it through a full six to eight hours without needing a nighttime potty run. Before we discuss how normal bladder conditions become impeded, a look at the design of our plumbing will be helpful.

Look Out Below!

When it comes to how we produce and eliminate urine, both sexes have pretty much the same hardware. The kidneys are responsible for filtering waste and excess water out of the bloodstream. Urine, which has been manufactured by the kidneys, travels "south" through a pair of flexible pipes called the *ureters* (one from the left kidney and one from the right). The ureters deposit the yellow stuff directly into the awaiting bladder, which can be likened to a muscular sack (see figure 5.1). The bladder stores this collected urine until it expands to the point where it feels compelled to send your brain the message "It's time to go!" And when your bladder reaches that stage (or when it thinks it has reached it), it will begin to cramp until it wakes you up so it can be emptied—usually in a hurry.

Both men's and women's bladders are connected to the outside world by one final piece of flexible pipe called the *urethra* (a term confusingly close to *ureter,* which we defined above). In males, the urethra runs the length of the penis, and in females the urethra ends at the front (anterior) aspect of the vagina.

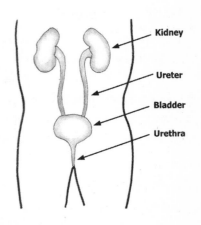

The primary structure holding back urine is a small muscular *sphincter* or valve located between the floor of the bladder and the top of the urethra (again, see figure 5.1). The sphincter and bladder receive additional physical support from the muscular

FIGURE 5.1

floor of the pelvis, which is made up of individual muscles whose names would take too long to type!

When something goes awry in this delicately regulated voiding system, urine will leak out when it should have stayed in—or else it will bring new meaning to the phrase "Gotta run!"

If all your plumbing is in working order, you should find yourself urinating *five to eight times a day.* That's about every two to five daytime hours.[3] (Drinking caffeinated or alcoholic beverages or taking diuretic medication will increase this frequency, as mentioned earlier.) Each time you empty your bladder, your urine stream should be strong, and it should last for ten or more seconds. Those who suffer from *nocturia,* or nighttime excursions to the toilet , will find themselves visiting the bathroom far more than eight times per day.

And when they do begin to relieve themselves, they may find their urine stream to be weak, the duration of urination lasting less than ten seconds (probably more like five or six), or both. These folks are likely dealing with some form of *incontinence*. (Although the term may conjure up the image of a full-out pants-wetting, it simply means the involuntary loss of urine—if only just a drop or two.)

Describing Incontinence

Before we dive into discussing potential cures for various plumbing problems, let's define the five types of urinary incontinence and their underlying causes. This way you'll be able to accurately describe your condition when visiting your physician. Once we home in on what may be wrong with your internal plumbing, then we can discuss treatment options to restore uninterrupted nights of sleep.

#1: Stress Incontinence

One day you are laughing so hard, you literally wet your pants— a wee little bit. Next you begin to notice yourself instinctively squeezing your knees together when you sneeze or cough to prevent or lessen urine leakage. Wetness that started off rare has now become regular. *Stress incontinence* (physical stress, not emotional stress) plagues far more women than is accounted for in statistics, because of the embarrassment involved.

The underlying cause of this problem is a straightforward plumbing issue. There is a leaky valve. The bladder's sphincter has become weakened. In addition to this muscular ring loosening, the muscles that make up your pelvic floor are likely deconditioned, stretched out, or unresponsive. Given this lack of support, when your abdominal muscles contract hard against your bladder, as is the case with sneezing, coughing, or laughing, or during heavy lifting, urine gets squeezed out—no matter how hard you squeeze your knees together.

As a physical therapist, I always question my patients about urine leakage. The reason is because low-back pain is very much related to weakened *core muscles*—of which the pelvic floor muscles are a key part. Shortly I will detail an important exercise that I teach to my patients, which helps restore the needed strength. Diligently retraining your pelvic-floor muscles can put an end to stress incontinence within a week.

#2: Urge Incontinence

Also known as the "overactive bladder," *urge incontinence* is the primary culprit in nighttime bathroom runs—and will therefore be the focus of the remainder of this chapter. If your bladder is under pressure from abnormal conditions, such as crowding from displaced pelvic organs (in women) or excessive growth of existing pelvic organs (both women and men), it will not have the space to fill fully.

During the day the overactive bladder will present itself at key times. The first is known literally as "key-in-the-lock" syndrome. People who are plagued by urge incontinence, as soon as they get home and put their key in the door lock, will suddenly experience an urgent need to use the toilet. Other life situations that get the overactive bladder going include standing up from a seated position, drinking a beverage and—interestingly—listening to running water. It appears that this problem has a conditioned side to it as well. If all this is ringing true with you, you may want to think twice about installing that waterfall decoration near your patio!

#3: Overflow Incontinence

With *overflow incontinence*, the bladder is filled to capacity and is simply running over. People struggling with this have difficulty starting their urine stream, and tend to have a weakened stream when they do get it going. These problems hamper their ability to sufficiently empty their bladder. So they find they must use the bathroom again, and again, and again in order to stay dry. And whenever they try to stretch out the time between trips to the toilet, overflow dripping begins once more. Most such sufferers have become well aware of the benefit of protective absorption pads to insure them against "water damage."

#4: Functional Incontinence

Found mostly in persons with physical handicaps, *functional incontinence* exists because the physical process of getting to the bathroom, disrobing to use the toilet, or both are too difficult and the person simply can't make it there in time. Frustratingly, this incontinence happens en route to the toilet. This problem is lessened by not waiting too long after you first get the message from your brain that your bladder is uncomfortable. Also, by wearing uncomplicated clothes, a person with arthritis or other physical limitations won't get caught short. (Dress for success here. No belts, suspenders, or buttoned and zippered pants, and of course, no overalls.)

#5: Mixed Incontinence

Mixed incontinence is one part stress incontinence and one part urge incontinence. This condition, sadly, is quite commonplace, especially in women over 50.

If you are going to get back into a routine of sleeping straight through the night, then you'll need to identify if there is a specific structural reason why your overactive bladder behaves the way it does.

Here's Where We Must Part Ways

While both sexes have the same basic urinary hardware and have similar struggles with nocturia, the dissimilar layout of the surrounding pelvic structures creates our unique male and female plumbing issues. That being the case, let's launch into separate discussions of sex-specific causes and cures.

For Men Only

When it comes to increased frequency of nighttime urination in men, we often need to look no further than the prostate gland. This gland, unique to men, sits just below the bladder, surrounding the most internal part of the urethra (see figure 5.2).

The prostate gland was designed to produce some of the support fluid that mixes with a man's sperm prior to ejaculation. Normally the size of a walnut, the prostate gland almost always enlarges to some degree as men grow older—particularly after

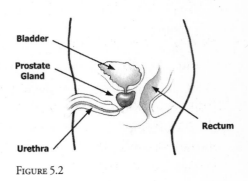

Figure 5.2

the age of 50. However, if this gland grows to the point of occupying too much pelvic real estate, it will begin to put the squeeze on the bladder.

In medical terms, the enlargement of the prostate is known as *benign prostatic hypertrophy*, or BPH. When in a grossly enlarged state, the prostate gland can partially obstruct the urethra as well, which leads to urine stream changes. Fortunately, less than half of men with BPH show symptoms. The ones who do might experience one or more of the following:[4]

- dribbling at the end of urinating
- inability to urinate (urinary retention)
- incomplete emptying of the bladder
- incontinence
- pain with urination or bloody urine (these may indicate infection)
- slowed or delayed start of the urinary stream

- straining to urinate
- strong and sudden urge to urinate
- weak urine stream
- needing to urinate two or more times per night

If you have one or more of these symptoms and are waking repeatedly to urinate, plan a visit to a urologist, whose specialty includes the evaluation and treatment of BPH. If your doctor determines that your prostate gland is indeed enlarged (noted via a digital rectal exam or an ultrasound test), he or she will typically order a blood test to check your *PSA,* or *prostate specific antigen* level (to rule out any sinister causes for the enlargement). If your PSA value is only slightly high, your doctor will likely take a wait-and-see approach, monitoring your PSA levels periodically.

HEALTHY PROSTATE GROWTH CYCLE[5]

Life stage	Weight in grams
Birth	1.5 grams
Puberty	11 grams
Mid-20s	18 grams
50s to 70s	18 grams → 31 grams
Unhealthy Prostate = 50 to 100 grams	

It has long been recognized that a significantly elevated PSA can be indicative of prostate cancer, which is best caught—as with all cancers—earlier, rather than later. So if your PSA level is deemed high this could warrant further medical evaluation, such as a biopsy of the prostate gland itself, followed by a CT scan or MRI and possibly even a bone scan (if other tests have started to wave a medical red flag).

Sadly, one in six men will be diagnosed with prostate cancer at some point during their lifetime.[6] The incidence of this diagnosis increases with age—starting in the forties and especially beyond the age of 65.[7] However, medical advances in both the diagnosis of and intervention for prostate cancer have made the treatment of this disease (especially in its early stages) quite successful—significantly enhancing the longevity of those affected. So if you have any of the BPH symptoms bulleted above do not delay in getting yourself in for a checkup.

If, on the upside, tests have deemed you cancer-free, yet your prostate's overgrowth is problematic, your urologist might prescribe the medication Proscar (generic, finasteride) in a moderate to severe case, or the natural supplement saw palmetto for a milder case. Both of these treatments work to shrink an overgrown prostate gland, which will significantly reduce the squeezing effect on your bladder. (*Note:* The positive effects of saw palmetto remain inconsistently supported in research studies.) When saw palmetto is prescribed, the recommended dosage is typically 320 milligrams per day. Before taking any supplement, discuss it with your doctor first. Wouldn't it be wonderful if one of these two pills was all you needed to sleep through the night again?

For Women Only

The first time I got on a trampoline after the birth of my children, I felt as if my intestines were going to drop through the floor of my pelvis. As a former gymnast, that really caught me by surprise. Three jumps into it and I felt compelled to use the ladies' room before my bouncy aerobics class got underway!

The physical stress of pregnancy and vaginal delivery really takes a toll on the female pelvis, and it seems to become worse as time wears on. Urinary incontinence, to some degree, will affect most women who have gone the route of childbearing, and even some of those who haven't. I say "to some degree" because, remember, urinary incontinence is simply the involuntary loss of urine—regardless of the amount. Even a few drops during a big sneeze or a belly laugh will grant you membership into this not-so-exclusive group.

As women, we usually head to our gynecologists when we have toileting troubles—after all, they *are* the doctor of "down there." While this is certainly appropriate, your general physician is also a good starting place, as is a urologist, whose specialty includes the treatment of women with urinary dysfunction. Whichever medical path you choose, it will help you to look at the unique feminine whys behind your woes—so you will be better prepared for upcoming conversations.

What makes women so susceptible to urge and stress incontinence? After all, we don't even have a prostate gland to contend with. Well, first of all, our pelvic neighborhoods are very crowded. Our vital female structures are lined up right next to each other in a way that doesn't allow much room for mobility and expansion. Not only are we packing the equipment to urinate and defecate, but we are also designed to carry and deliver live young!

Second, the foundation of our pelvis (the muscular floor) takes a beating, particularly during pregnancy and vaginal delivery, or when supporting an oversized load of belly fat. When that foundation begins to sag, some of the structures that should be located on the "second floor" drop down to the first—and on occasion plummet straight through to the basement. Here is where a few pictures will be worth, quite literally, a thousand words.

Cystocele. The most widespread pelvic problem that aging women face is typically referred to as a "dropped bladder," but more technically as a *cystocele* (see figure 5.3). When the muscular sling, or hammock, that holds your internal pelvic organs in place begins to weaken, there will be a southern shift in the position of your bladder. This move downward will put increased pressure on the sphincter (valve) between the bladder and the urethra. In addition, the bladder will begin to *recline*—pushing into and deforming the front wall of your vagina. (Sometimes this bulge can be felt when one is wiping after urination.)

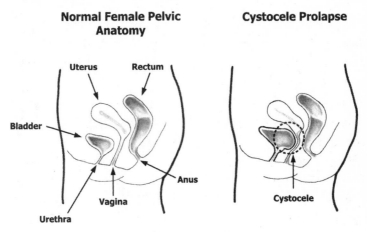

Normal Female Pelvic Anatomy   **Cystocele Prolapse**

FIGURE 5.3

Many factors feed into this condition. Menopause and aging can be added to the previously mentioned stressors of pregnancy, childbirth, and overweight. But there are a number of possible fixes—one for mild-to-moderate incontinence issues and a few others for severe problems. We will discuss each of them below.

Uterine prolapse. Another condition some women will face is a "falling uterus." The uterus can actually begin to drop down into the vagina (see figure 5.4), and in severe cases it can actually protrude through the vaginal opening. Just as with a cystocele, a fallen uterus will create extra bladder pressure, not allowing it its full expansion capacity. Again, the primary culprit is a weakened pelvic floor. (Are you beginning to see a recurring theme here?) When advanced and problematic, a prolapsed uterus calls for a surgical remedy, which we will discuss in the treatment section below.

Rectocele. Finally, structurally produced urge incontinence in

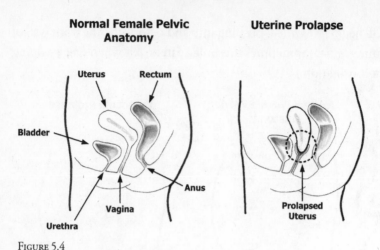

FIGURE 5.4

women can stem from a weakened rectal wall, which allows the rectum (and its fecal contents) to bulge against the vagina. Subsequently, like falling dominos, the vagina is pushed against the back of the bladder (see figure 5.5). Once again, deconditioned pelvic-floor muscles play a role in this collapse. (Chronic constipation, which leads to stool impaction in the lower portion of the bowel, can have the same squeezing effect on the bladder as the rectal prolapse or rectocele does. So—fiber, water, fiber, water...enough said.)

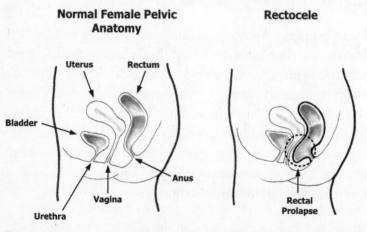

FIGURE 5.5

Here's the good news, though. The crowding your bladder may be experiencing doesn't need to be permanent. Problems such as those mentioned above can be treated effectively and, many times, noninvasively, so you can get back to sleeping soundly. Here's how:

Conquering Your Overactive Bladder

The self-treatments I feature below, as well as the pharmaceutical intervention noted, are for both men and women. What's good for the goose is good for the gander. When situations increase in severity to the point of requiring surgery, the two sexes again part ways. In a word, however, there is much that can be done.

Retrain Your Pelvic Floor

Deconditioned pelvic-floor muscles are incapable of tightening (contracting) adequately. When you sneeze, cough, or laugh, they should automatically tighten up extra hard to resist against the increased internal pressure. Also, whenever we are standing, or when we must strain to do something, we need the natural support these muscles were designed to bring. When they quit bringing it, things begin to "swing low, sweet chariot…"

When the bottom has dropped out of your pelvic support system, it's time to spring into action. As with any other flabby muscle group, they likely need to be retrained. And I have just the right exercise for you. Now, you don't need to break a sweat here. You don't even need to join a gym or buy a yoga mat. *Kegel exercises* can be performed anytime and anywhere, and nobody needs to know. Here's how the procedure goes:

1. Inhale normally and pause.

2. Tighten up the muscles around your rectum as if you were holding back the urge to have a bowel movement.

3. Maintain that squeezing contraction while exhaling.

4. Continue to breathe in and out for a cycle of 10 breaths while maintaining your tightened bottom. (If you can't hold the contraction for 10 breath cycles, begin with 10 repetitions of however many breath cycles you can hold through—even if it is just one.)

5. Repeat 10 times. Do this 3 to 5 times during the day.

If you regularly perform this exercise, you may notice changes in your stress and urge incontinence by the end of the week!

Bathroom Behavior Modification

An overactive bladder, by nature, will prompt more bathroom runs than you'd like. The problem with visiting the bathroom so frequently is that you are most likely voiding before your bladder is truly full (as would be demonstrated by a urine stream which lasts less than ten seconds). When this behavior pattern is followed throughout the day, it doesn't call it quits just because it's nighttime. Basically, your bladder has been taught bad habits.

A bladder-retraining method called *scheduled voiding* is very effective. Gradually, you increase the time between bathroom runs until you regain the ability to tolerate just eight per day. So, for instance, if you feel the need to urinate every 30 minutes, try stretching that out to 35 or 40 minutes. Increase this by 5-minute intervals until you reach normal (basically every two hours).

Another behavior modification that will aid the retraining process is to quit emptying your bladder every time you get ready to leave the house—just in case. If you don't have a ten-second urine stream, you may have jumped the gun. With both of these changes, you are working to restore more stretch (and capacity) to your bladder before it begins to cry out.

Medications

Prescription medicines that target the bladder can be real quality-of-life-savers. *Anticholinergic* medications decrease bladder contractions (therefore decreasing the urge to void). They have an added bonus of increasing one's bladder capacity, due to the lengthened time they allow between toileting. As with most prescription drugs there are side effects, such as dry mouth and eyes, constipation, and headaches. Yet most people will choose these over a hyperactive bladder.

Below is a list of some commonly prescribed medications on the market today.

Prescription medications designed to treat the overactive bladder:

- Detrol LA
- Ditropan XL (also Oxytrol and Gelnique)
- Enablex
- Sanctura
- Vesicare

Pessaries: For Women Only

A *pessary* is a removable, ring-shaped plastic or silicone device that is placed into the vagina and acts as a structural support for those pesky, fallen pelvic organs. For some, the use of a pessary is all that is required to relieve their problem. Others may find that a pessary can hold off the need for surgery for many years—which is a good thing.

Surgery

For men with urinary incontinence caused by advanced BPH, a partial removal of the prostate is often necessary. This procedure acts to remove the urine stream obstruction. The surgical approach is either through the lower abdomen or via the urethra (through the penis).

Women who have incontinence due to a significantly shifted bladder, uterus, or rectum will also benefit from targeted gynecological or rectal surgeries. *Bladder* and *uterine lift procedures* commonly use a mesh sling to mimic the action of the once-supportive pelvic-floor muscles. This sling, when sewn into place, restores the bladder or uterus to its original position. In the case of a severely prolapsed uterus, a partial or full hysterectomy (removal of the uterus or the ovaries and uterus) may be warranted. Surgical correction of a rectocele that has been unresponsive to dietary changes (remember: fiber, water, fiber, water) can be performed either through the anus or the vagina, between the two, or from the abdomen above.

According to the National Association for Continence, nearly 200,000 surgeries for pelvic organ prolapse (POP) are performed annually in the U.S. alone. This means approximately 11 percent of women will have surgery for POP or urinary incontinence by age 80. Unfortunately, nearly 30 percent of these women will need another surgery due to failure or because of recurrence of prolapse or treatment of another, often related pelvic-floor problem.[8] As my Jewish grandmother would have said, *Oy! It's tough being a woman!*

As we have seen in this chapter, your nighttime trips to the toilet are not just "the way things are now." There is so much you can do to help—even before you have to venture to the doctor's office. For those of you with more advanced incontinence issues, let me encourage you again that partnering with a specialized medical professional can do wonders for recapturing your beauty sleep!

Now on to the next sleep-stealer…pain.

Chapter 6

Painfully Awake

Say Good Night to Your Body's Aches and Pains

Over the years I've treated two types of patients. In the first group are those whose bodies' aches and pains gnaw at them during the day, but finally quit when they lie down at night. The second group is typically the most frustrated, however. Even though they drop into bed at the end of the day, exhausted and in much need of some healing sleep, their body just won't allow them that luxury. These folks have little respite from pain because, even when they do fall asleep, they are repeatedly awakened during the night.

Here's a fascinating fact that Dr. Lee Shangold, otolaryngologist (ENT) and board-certified sleep specialist, shared with me: Chronic pain disrupts your regular sleep cycles even while you're still asleep. How can your sleep be interrupted if you are still asleep? In chapter 2, we discussed how the brain's alpha waves are normally present fully when we are awake and to a lesser degree in N1, the drifting-off-to-sleep phase and in the dream, or REM, phase.

Interestingly, sleep studies of people who suffer from chronic pain show that alpha (alert) brain waves pop up repeatedly throughout the deeper phases of sleep (N2 and N3). These out-of-place waves are unwelcome interruptions to what should be the most physically healing portions of your sleep cycle. No wonder you can't get well!

Sometimes all that stands between you and a good night's sleep is a subtle change in the placement of your head and limbs. By altering sleeping posture, many people can absolutely silence their body's pain signals. Over the past twenty or so years I have helped thousands of patients to get their nocturnal pain to settle down so they, too, can settle down for the night.

Rick was one of those patients. He had been losing sleep for months because of a painful shoulder. He couldn't lie on it—the pain was way too sharp. And when he lay on his back or on his other side his shoulder just throbbed. During his initial evaluation I gave him some quick instruction in altering his sleeping posture and pillow setup. The next visit he was all smiles. He had clocked two full nights of sleep—and I had yet to "treat" him.

Each fix I offer in this chapter is going to address your lying-down posture, your pillows, and the positioning of one or more parts of your body. Everyone's body needs to be adequately supported while they sleep, and in the case of a painful joint, bursa, muscle, or disc-related problem this need for support becomes crucial. At times I will refer to "filling up the negative space." By this I mean bringing a supportive surface up to meet the body at each of its raised curves—the empty (negative) spaces between your body parts and your bed. An example is adequately filling up the negative space in between your neck and your pillow in the side-lying sleeping position (the space that is present because of the width of your shoulders).

You will soon discover that if you position yourself better at night, you can ease (and possibly even silence) your body's pain signals. Not only will this allow you to spend more time sleeping, but you will also benefit by not having your non-REM brain-wave patterns interrupted all night. I truly hope that after reading through this chapter you will have found a sleeping posture tailor-made for your condition. Then, even tonight, you may finally be able to secure the kind of healing sleep your body has been longing for.

Head, Shoulders, Knees, and Toes...

Did you sing this song when you were a kid? Back then it never occurred to us that we were pointing out all the places our future aches and pains would reside! When your extremities are in an irritable mood, you are not going to fall asleep—not for a while, at least. Sometimes they may allow you to *initiate* sleep, but then they rudely wake you in the middle of the night demanding attention. Let's deal with those sleep-disruptive body parts first.

Headaches

For over two decades I have been successfully freeing patients from chronic head pain—without medication. Frustrated for years with traditional medicine's approach to its treatment (*Take this pill, then that shot...*), in 2008 I finally wrote a book titled *Overcoming Headaches and Migraines*. After helping the reader gain a better understanding of the cause and effect of their condition, I present a step-by-step, tried-and-true method of curing, rather than simply managing, persistent head pain. The ability to enable so many people to live pain-free and medication-free has been my great joy.

Part of my approach to eliminating head pain is to address the negative influences of harmful postures. Again and again, simple postural changes can relieve a significant percentage of head pain—before I even start hands-on treatment. On occasion, postural change is the only intervention needed.

One of the postures I always need to address in the head-pain sufferer is the spatial relationship between their head and their pillow. Let me take you through a few scenarios based on the positions you find yourself sleeping in.*

---

* For photographs of each posture described in this section, visit my website at www.LisaMorrone .com, Free Resources/Sleeping Postures, or refer to my books *Overcoming Back and Neck Pain* or *Overcoming Headaches and Migraines*.

1. Side-lying. In this position it is crucial for the bridge of your nose to be in line with (parallel to) your breastbone, as it is when you're standing. Any angle between the two, either because your head is propped up too high or has dropped down too low, will cause your neck to side-bend. This tipped-up or dropped-down position will provoke head pain by stressing your headache-producing neck components (for example, muscles, discs, joints). In order to sleep in a posture that won't aggravate pain, depending on how large your shoulders are, you may need to sleep on a flat pillow, a fluffy one, or possibly on two pillows. The goal is the same for everyone here—the bridge of your nose must be in line with your breastbone.

2. Back-lying. It's essential to make sure your head and neck structures are in a neutral position throughout the night—not bent forward or backward. The best way is to use just enough pillow support under your head to keep your head in the same plane as your shoulders (just as it is when you are standing). This neutral alignment will neutralize the noxious stress that sleeping with your head in a forward- or backward-bent position places on sensitive areas. If you are unsure of your alignment, have someone look at you when you lie down. Then adjust your pillow height according to their input and these rules.

3. Stomach-lying. Let me say this for the first time in this book— but not the last time—*do not sleep on your stomach* if you have headaches. This could very well be the reason you have head pain. Stomach-sleeping (or prone lying) is a very mechanically damaging position for the discs and joints in your neck, and for the muscles that connect your head to your neck.

A body pillow is a great help for those of you trying to kick the habit of stomach-sleeping:

1. Run the pillow between your legs and in front of your chest.

2. Roll forward onto the pillow and slide your bottom leg back behind you a bit so only your top leg is in contact with the pillow.

3. Allow your face to slip slightly off the side edge of the regular pillow that is under your head. (This will keep the rotation of your neck to a minimum).

Nothing good comes from sleeping on your stomach—in my practice I often get to treat the lifetime offenders.

EVEN MIGRAINES MAY RESPOND POSITIVELY TO A BETTER SETUP

Migraine headaches are experienced by people whose brains are extra sensitive to noxious input. Migraineurs have lowered *headache thresholds*—the stimulus point at which their head pain begins.

The pain-onset threshold of a migraine is typically reached after a number of irritants (triggers) have piled up on one another. These trigger can include loud noise, food sensitivities, bright lights, strong odors, hormone swings, and most typically, I've found, upper-neck dysfunction. If you sleep in a position that irritates the pain-sensitive structures in your neck, then you are ensuring that the upper-neck trigger remains a constant. By removing just that one component, you may find that your other triggers can no longer pile high enough to reach your head-pain threshold. Now wouldn't that be a bonus?

Shoulder Pain

There are many reasons why your shoulder may be causing you some discomfort. However, when the pain begins to wake you up from a sound sleep, you know you have a serious problem. Common shoulder diagnoses include bursitis, tendonitis, impingement syndrome, and frozen shoulder (adhesive capsulitis).

If you have had surgery to repair your rotator cuff or shave off a bit of your *acromion* (the bony "roof" sitting above your shoulder socket), or another invasive procedure, then you know that sleeping comfortably is a challenge.

Then there is the misleading kind of pain that absolutely feels as if it were emanating from your shoulder joint, but is actually due to a compressed nerve or degenerated disc in your neck. Whatever is causing your pain, here's some professional advice to soothe that sore shoulder of yours so you can rest better and heal faster:

1. Side-lying. If your right shoulder is the problem, you've already figured out that you should avoid sleeping on your right side. When you are lying on your pain-free side, it is extremely important to support your painful arm with a pillow or two (depending on your trunk width). This pillow setup is often most comfortable when placed directly in front of your chest, though some people find that if there is some pillow support (or even a folded hand towel) between their upper arm and rib cage (in the region of your armpit), they are much more comfortable. Try it tonight—you may finally be able to sleep comfortably despite the bursitis or tendonitis that you are dealing with.

2. Back-lying. When you lie on your back, your arms must drop somewhat behind your neutral arm position in order to meet your mattress. This position of the shoulder is called *extension*, and even though it measures only 10 to 20 degrees for most body types, it's enough to irritate the pain sources within your shoulder. Your arm reacts by sending out a constant stream of pain signals to your brain—which is far more effective at waking you up than any alarm clock you own. A quick fix is to place a folded towel or small flat pillow alongside your trunk. When your arm lies down beside you it is then protected from having to spend the night in extension.

3. Stomach-lying. Again, not a good choice. There is no healthy (pain-free) place to put your arm when you are lying facedown. The shoulder joint always loses.

Knee Pain

Aging knees…they are painful when you're upright and achy when you lie still. Most knee problems come with a side of edema, which is swelling located within the knee joint itself. A swollen knee would rather avoid the extreme end ranges of knee motion—full *flexion*, or bending, and full *extension*, or complete straightening. In other words, cranky knees like a gentle bend. That is the factor you must pay attention to when positioning yourself for sleep if knee pain is your issue.

1. Side-lying. If you sleep best on your side, then you are in luck, because your knees are usually slightly bent when doing so. Here's an extra bit of comfort: Place one pillow lengthwise between your legs—from your inner thigh to your lower leg. This decreases the direct pressure of one knee resting on top of the other. Most often you will find you are more comfortable if your troublesome knee is on the top side (the one nearest the ceiling). Also, try to keep your knees bent to only about 30 degrees. With that amount of bend you'll have the most anatomical space between your lower and upper leg bones (at your knee joint).

2. Back-lying. While you are on your back, simply place a pillow under your knees to maintain a gentle bend in them for the purpose of increasing their internal joint space, and therefore your comfort. Try placing the pillow in both the horizontal and vertical orientations—often one works better than the other depending on the individual.

3. Stomach-lying. As you are likely beginning to understand, stomach-lying is not good for *any* part of your body. That said, if nothing else hurts you at this time and you are a dedicated belly sleeper, try placing a pillow under the tops of your feet so your knee remains slightly bent. Better yet, train yourself to adopt another position.

Toe Pain

Your toes are made up of 19 small bones and 14 joints, or junction points. It is highly important that all those moving parts maintain their mobility if you are to get the most out of them. Your two feet take quite a beating. When you walk, your full body weight is transferred to one foot at a time. When you run—if you run—each foot must absorb upward of three to four times the weight of your body. All day, every day, your feet get stepped on mercilessly—especially if you are overweight. Therefore, over time you may find that you're beginning to develop painful arthritis in your toes.

In this society, our ten toes are typically jammed into footwear for a large part of our waking hours. When you take those tired dogs out of your shoes and put them in bed, they may begin to throb or ache.

Your best preventive action is to soak your feet in very warm water for 10 to 20 minutes before bedtime. Since arthritis loves heat, soaking allows that warmth to encircle each toe joint. Follow up with a gentle massage of your tootsies (use some moisturizing cream on your hands for ease of glide). Next, slowly and carefully bend every toe knuckle forward (flex) and back (extend) about five to ten times, and then side to side (this applies only to the joints that separate your toes from the meaty part of your foot). This prebedtime routine will give your toes the attention they need so they won't have to clamor for it when you turn out the lights.

PAIN IN A LOWER LIMB THAT COMES FROM YOUR BACK

Sometimes pain that you believe to be originating from your hip, thigh, knee, calf, or foot is actually *referred pain* from your lower-back region. Referred, or *radicular*, pain is pain that migrates out from a more central pain source. The most typical leg-pain-referring structures are the lumbar discs and the sciatic nerve (a bundle of spinal nerves which cross under your buttock muscles and run down the back of your leg).

If your daytime leg symptoms are worse when you're sitting than when standing or walking, this is a strong sign that your back is to blame for your nighttime limb pain. In this case, a visit to a spine specialist—an orthopedist, a manual physical therapist, or a medical doctor whose specialty area is orthopedics—is strongly recommended.

Soothing Your Spine

Back and neck pain are extremely common and tremendously life-altering. So much is lost—sleep, wages, recreational activities… even the simplest of everyday functions are difficult to complete in some cases. Throughout my career I have helped people in restoring their spines to full health. In early 2008 I published my first book, *Overcoming Back and Neck Pain*, to enable readers to gain control over their own pain by learning to treat it themselves. That book is sold all over the world, and I have received many wonderful success stories. I am thrilled to have the opportunity to have a healing touch far beyond that of my own private practice and my college classroom.

As with the treatment of head pain, a significant component of recovering from spine pain has to do with how we position ourselves. Sleeping posture is absolutely critical for healing and to avoid ongoing injury. When seeking the best position for your spine to rest in, you must pay attention to its overall alignment. Your hurting spine is happiest when it is in a neutral position—not excessively side-bent, rotated, bent forward, or bent backward.

Back Pain

Whether you have acute or chronic back pain, you need to get yourself as much sleep as you can. Sleep heals—it's as simple as that.

Here's great news: You can sleep more comfortably tonight, and even possibly wake up pain-free, just by following my advice about your sleeping posture.* So let's try to get you some more sleep!

1. Side-lying. If you sleep on your side without properly supporting your top leg and top arm, then you will naturally rotate your spine forward until those limbs come into contact with the bed. Also, without leg support, some people draw both of their knees up into a fetal position. This creates too much bending, or flexion, of the lower (lumbar) spine. The other harmful option in an unsupported side-lying position is to bend your top hip and draw your top knee up high while straightening the other leg (sort of like a frog-leg position on one side). This forces your spine to remain in a rotated position all night long. Even if you keep both of your legs relatively straight, without the necessary support of your top leg your spine will settle into a side-bent position because of the width of your hips and shoulders.

Maintaining a happy and healthy spine position means avoiding excessive flexion, rotation, and side-bending. Here's where a body pillow comes in very handy. Simply place the lower half of the body pillow between your slightly bent legs and use the top half in front of your chest to support your top arm. If you don't have a body pillow, you can substitute two regular-length pillows. First lie on your preferred side and slip one pillow lengthwise between your legs from the groin area down to your lower leg. Next add the second pillow lengthwise in front of your trunk so you can rest your top arm on it.

2. Back-lying. Not too much can go wrong in this position, provided your mattress is still supportive enough to prevent you from sinking down into the bed hammock-style. (On that note, it is a good idea to replace a traditional mattress every ten years.) In order to give your back an even better rest position, place a pillow

---

* For photographs of each posture described in this section, visit my website at www.LisaMorrone .com, Free Resources/Sleeping Postures, or refer to my book *Overcoming Back and Neck Pain*.

lengthwise under the backs of your legs, placing one end just below your buttock crease. This will keep much of the weight of your legs from pulling on your low back. It accomplishes this by placing your hip's joints in a position of ease (slight flexion), which allows the hip muscles that connect to your spine to relax.

3. Stomach-lying. I told you I would begin to sound like a broken record here. By maintaining your on-the-belly position of relative extension (slight backward bending of the spine) all night, you are preventing the back portion of your discs (the part that usually bulges or ruptures) from healing and receiving the nourishment they need. Additionally, in this non-neutral posture your spine's joints are compressed—which is never good for the conditions of arthritis or stenosis (the narrowing of the bony canals through which your spinal cord or spinal nerves run).

Here's my suggestion for reform: Get hold of a body pillow. Set it up just as I described above in the side-lying section. Then roll forward onto the pillow and slide your bedside leg back behind you some so only your top leg is in contact with the pillow. (This modification has allowed about 80 percent of my staunch stomach-sleeping patients to kick their bad-for-the-back habit.)

HOW ONE PILLOW SAVED A WOMEN'S MINISTRY

Two years ago I received a letter from a very grateful reader. This woman began by describing her six-month battle with back and leg pain. It had gotten so bad that she even had trouble putting on her shoes in the morning. Yet the most troubling thing for her was that she was unable to sit long enough to read and study her Bible each morning; her leg pain was just too intense. At the time she found my book *Overcoming Back and Neck Pain*, she told me she was seriously considering resigning from her leadership position in the flourishing women's ministry she had developed years earlier, all because of her inability to sit and prepare her materials.

Desperate, this reader stood in order to read my book. She excitedly explained that by chapter 3 (the posture chapter) she had stumbled upon something that was, in her own words, "unbelievable." She read my advice about using a pillow under her legs when she slept on her back—which she had already been doing. However, I had recommended that the pillow be placed *lengthwise, along* the backs of her legs, rather than just crosswise under her knees.

The very first morning she was surprised to awake with less pain. Putting on her shoes was easier. By day three the unbelievable happened—her pain was completely gone! She could put her shoes on, sit to study, and resume all her daily responsibilities, all without a return of her pain. She told me I might not believe that this had happened...but then she corrected herself and said that I probably would since I had been giving this same advice to my patients for over 20 years.

She was right—I did believe her. It's often the subtle changes that make the most difference. I was so encouraged when she closed her e-mail by telling me her ability to minister to other women could now continue unhindered!

Neck Pain

Earlier I mentioned the concept of filling up the negative space when you lie down to sleep. This goal is ultra-important when you are attempting to ease your pain in the neck. A neck that is left hanging down toward your pillow, or that is propped up too high all night, is going to begin complaining sooner or later. If you treat your neck to just the right amount of support, it will pipe down and let you sleep.

If you read the earlier section on head pain, you will notice that I basically reiterate what I recommended there. Why? Because the goal here is identical: a nearly neutral head and neck position.*

---

* Again, for photographs of each posture described in this section, visit my website: www.LisaMor rone.com, Free Resources/Sleeping Postures, or refer to my book *Overcoming Back and Neck Pain.*

1. Side-lying. When you're on your side it is crucial for the bridge of your nose to stay in line with your breastbone, as it is when you are standing. Any angle or tilt between these two bony structures because your head is too high or too low will cause your neck to side-bend. Sleeping night after night in a non-neutral position will place significant strain on the joints, discs, and any overtight muscles in your neck.

In order to relieve this strain, you may need to sleep on a flat pillow, a fluffy one, or possibly on two pillows depending on how large your shoulders are. Some people do well by adding further support at the nape of their necks with a rolled-up hand towel they slip lengthwise into the bottom edge of their pillowcase. This neck roll can be made smaller or larger depending on your comfort. The third suggestion I have, which makes a huge difference, is to sleep with your top arm resting on a large fluffy pillow placed in front of your chest. By supporting your arm and shoulder in this more neutral position, you will avoid bottom-up, trunk-into-neck rotation, which creates significant twisting at the base of your neck.

2. Back-lying. It's important for a person who suffers with nagging neck pain to make sure their head and neck structures are not bent forward or tipped backward too much. The best way is to use just enough pillow support under your head to make you look like you do when standing—your head aligned squarely over your shoulders. This will take undue stress off your pain-producing neck structures. If you are unsure of your alignment, have someone look at you when you lie down, then adjust your pillows according to these rules.

3. Stomach-lying. For the final time in this chapter, I will repeat my warning: *Do not sleep on your stomach* if you have neck pain. This may very well be the reason your neck has ended up causing you so much discomfort. As I explained in the head-pain section, when you lie on your belly, you force your neck to twist fully to one side so that you can breathe. This "screwed up" posture places the discs and joints in your neck in an extremely damaging position.

A body pillow is a great help for those of you trying to break the habit of stomach-sleeping. Here are the directions, once again, for proper propping in this modified stomach-sleeping position:

1. Run the pillow between your legs and in front of your chest.

2. Roll forward onto the pillow and slide your bottom leg back behind you a bit so only your top leg is in contact with the pillow.

3. Allow your face to slip slightly off the side edge of the regular pillow that is under your head. (This will keep the rotation of your neck to a minimum).

This setup will keep the top-down rotation of your neck to a minimum, while supporting your top arm and shoulder protects against neck rotation from the bottom up.

SPENDING A FORTUNE TO FIND COMFORT

An out-of-town friend of mine was really excited when she got her hands on my first book, *Overcoming Back and Neck Pain*. Unbeknownst to me, this friend had been waking for the past three years with a neck ache. It would gradually diminish, but never fully go away, during the day. Each morning, there it was again.

Over those years, my friend had bought a series of new pillows to try. When that didn't help, she convinced her husband to replace their mattress. This purchase set them back a few thousand dollars. Imagine her frustration (and his) when she woke that first week on her new mattress with her neck pain unrelieved.

Reading about the principles of postural alignment for the neck-pain sufferer, she tried the side-lying setup that very night. The next morning she woke to a world without neck pain! And the next morning, and the morning after that! When she told me what had happened, she was completely thrilled that she was no longer beginning each day with an aching neck…though she was a bit frustrated that she had spent thousands in pursuit of relief, and it was the $12 book that saved her neck.

Acid Reflux

"I've got the GERD," people proclaim. The first time I heard someone say that, it sounded to me like some sort of fungal growth. Not so. What they are describing is the reflux, or regurgitation, of stomach acid into their lower esophagus. *GERD* stands for *gastroesophageal reflux disorder*, but it is more commonly known as good ole heartburn, even though it doesn't have anything to do with the heart. But burn—yes, it does indeed burn.

If you've "got the GERD," then you realize that the closer to horizontal you get, the worse your symptoms become. This is what makes sleeping with acid reflux so very challenging. Likely your doctor has told you to sleep with your head and shoulders up on three pillows, but how's that working for your neck? Maybe you've found that you've just exchanged the pain in your chest for a big pain in your neck.

By changing the alignment of your pillows, you will achieve a position that is not only good for your GERD, but better on your neck. Rather than piling up three pillows perpendicular to your body under your head and shoulders, simply rotate the top pillow so it is parallel with your trunk. This way, it will support not only your head and shoulders, but your trunk as well. This keeps everything from your head to your waist in neutral alignment, which removes undue stress from your spine. Ahh…so much better.*

---

* For photographs of the posture described in this section, visit my website at www.LisaMorrone .com, Free Resources/Sleeping Postures, or refer to my book *Overcoming Back and Neck Pain*.

The world is such a better place after a restful night of sleep. If your body has been keeping you from getting one recently, a new day may be dawning for you—one in which even the sun shines brighter. The reason I put so much emphasis on my patients' sleeping posture is because they spend one-third of their day in that position. If you wake up feeling unwell, or even worse than you did when you went to bed the night before, something is amiss.

However, once you find the sleeping posture that works best for you, you'll feel better the morning after, and you'll have your sleep debt paid off in no time. There is only one thing left to say: *Bonne nuit et faites de beaux rêves, mes amis*—Good night and sweet dreams, my friends.

Chapter 7

The Sleep Apnea Emergency

Oxygen 9-1-1

Some of my most vivid memories from childhood are the noises my father would make while he slept. On weekends I could hear him through his bedroom door loud and clear. And when he fell asleep on the couch while watching sports (which happened often), the odd symphony of snores, snorts, and such was enough to send my brothers and me into full-out belly laughs. It seemed my father was always tired. I don't ever recall him looking bright-eyed and bushy-tailed. Back then I just assumed it was because he worked six days a week.

Furthermore, my mother would complain regularly about his noisy nighttime behavior. At times, she would even try to imitate the sounds he made. This, of course, would rub my dad the wrong way and he would retort, "I'm just exhausted, Eleanor—what do you want from me?" I guess she just wanted him to quiet down so she could sleep.

Just a few short decades ago snoring was viewed as no more than an annoying trait that some people had—men more than women—and most people attributed it to being overweight or not being able to breathe through your nose adequately. Cases of snoring and other nocturnal clatter had not yet been connected to the possibility of serious health concerns…beyond the obvious loss of sleep for the snorer's partner.

The field of sleep science is relatively new. Even though researchers began to study brain-wave activity of sleeping subjects as far back as 1929 (thanks to the invention of the EEG—see chapter 2), serious study of the sleep disturbance now known as *sleep apnea* didn't take off until the late 1960s. Sleep apnea is defined as *the episodic reduction in airflow, or cessation of breathing, while one sleeps*. More specifically, an apnea is deemed to have occurred when a person either stops breathing altogether, or takes less than 25 percent of a normal breath, for a period lasting 10 seconds or more.

The first successful medical intervention for sleep apnea wasn't developed until 1981, when Dr. Colin Sullivan of the University of Sydney in Australia introduced the *CPAP machine*. CPAP (pronounced *SEE-pap*) stands for *continuous positive airway pressure*. This device, which props open a person's airway by providing a continuous stream of air under pressure, remains the standard treatment for sleep apnea today (more on this machine later). Over the last three decades scientists have discovered a great deal more about the relationship between nighttime breathing patterns and our physical and mental health. Today we understand the highly deleterious effect that reduced oxygen (caused by halted breathing) has on the brain and the rest of the body—not to mention the impact it has on our longevity.

Here's a list of what we now know to be true. Those who have untreated sleep apnea have a

- 20 times greater risk of cardiovascular disease
- 15 times greater risk for motor vehicle accidents
- 10 times greater risk for stroke
- 3 times greater risk for death from heart attack or stroke (with severe obstructive sleep apnea)

- much greater risk of sudden death (while asleep or within a few hours of waking)

- higher injury rate on the job

If my parents and their doctors had had access to all this information back then, I expect my father would have received treatment for what I now recognize to have been sleep apnea. And likely he would not have died from sleep apnea–associated heart disease at the unripe age of 59.

SEVEN WARNING SIGNS OF AN OXYGEN EMERGENCY[1]

1. Excessive daytime sleepiness

2. Loud snoring

3. You are observed by another to stop breathing at times while you sleep

4. Abrupt awakening, gasping for breath

5. Regularly wake with a very dry mouth or sore throat

6. Experience headaches in the morning

7. Trouble staying asleep throughout the night

Breathless in Bed

If you wake each morning after what you perceive to be a full night's sleep and have to drag yourself out of bed and through the day—something is likely amiss. And if you sleep with a partner who is complaining, like my mother did, about all the noise you make and the irregular breathing patterns you have while you sleep, then you might have stumbled upon the primary barrier between you and a refreshing night's sleep—sleep apnea.

The problem with sleep apnea has less to do with the cacophony you make, and everything to do with how many times your airflow dips dramatically, or stops altogether, during the night. Sleep studies reveal that sleep-apnea patients have apnea episodes (and remember, these episodes have to last ten or more seconds to be considered such) anywhere from 5 to *over 100 times* per hour…throughout the entire night. The amazing thing is that people with sleep apnea don't realize when they have actually stopped breathing (though a small number do have a form of this disorder that causes them to awake gasping for air). Yet even if you are sound asleep, completely unaware of your plight, your body's "breathing commander" (in the brain's medulla region) never sleeps.

Equipped with highly sensitive blood-oxygen sensors, your body stands poised to spring into action, if need be, to jump-start your breathing. It's quite a remarkable cascade of events. Upon sensing that your oxygen level is falling (from not inhaling) and your carbon dioxide level is rising (from not exhaling), your brain sounds an alarm deep within. A 9-1-1 call is made, prompting your body's adrenal glands to release a stimulating dose of adrenaline (a.k.a. epinephrine). This immediately raises your blood pressure and your level of alertness, just enough to jolt you into taking a deep breath, which initiates a normal breathing pattern once more.

If you do have sleep apnea, there are a couple of serious ramifications you need to concern yourself with right off the bat.

1. Your brain and body are not getting a regular supply
   of oxygen throughout the night. (Think of it as
   intermittent suffocation.) Without adequate oxygen,
   your body will age more rapidly (due to the condition
   known as *oxidative stress*). And therefore, you run
   a much greater risk of developing a whole host of
   cardiovascular complications, such as high blood
   pressure, stroke, or heart attack.[2] These disease processes
   are the result of *endothelial damage*—damage to the

lining of your blood vessels—which occurs because of the stress of oxygen deprivation.

2. Even though you are not aware of being wakened, your sleeping cycles are constantly being interrupted. No wonder you always feel tired—you're getting mini wake-up calls all night long!

It is important to understand that not all sleep-apnea conditions stem from the same source. In fact there are three categories: *central sleep apnea; obstructive sleep apnea;* and *complex,* or *mixed, sleep apnea.* Let's take some time up front to understand them, and then we'll look at some of the latest self-help and medical approaches you can make use of.

Central Sleep Apnea

The "central" in central sleep apnea (CSA) indicates a problem within the brain itself, the hub of your central nervous system. In a healthy system, the brain doesn't forget to tell the lungs to breathe. However, with CSA, that is just what occurs. Frightening, isn't it? Though it's not a problem during the daytime, somehow the brain's signal transmission halts repeatedly at night—and so does your breathing, if you suffer from CSA. Thank goodness for the backup breathing generator in your brain, which jolts you into taking an emergency breath. This form of sleep apnea, which is much less common, has been attributed primarily to underlying heart disease, previous stroke, narcotic usage, or brain tumor history.

Obstructive Sleep Apnea

Obstructive sleep apnea (OSA) affects nearly 18 million in the United States and is most frequently seen in overweight men.[3] As its name implies, the underlying cause is a physical obstruction, or blockage, in the upper airway. It most typically results from decreased tone in the muscles surrounding the throat. When a person with

OSA is relaxed (asleep) and reclined (lying down) this less-than-adequate muscle tone allows the soft palate (the back-end portion of the roof of the mouth) and other surrounding structures to collapse into the throat. This condition becomes more pronounced as you pass through the sleep cycle since with each successive phase you lose more and more muscle tone. The greatest trouble takes place during the REM phase, due to the fact that all the body's muscles become paralyzed (minus your heart, diaphragm, and eye muscles).

Other oral features that can create obstruction are enlarged tonsils or adenoids, or a large, fleshy uvula (the dangling object at the back of your mouth)—though obstructive adenoids are rarely an issue in adults, with the exception of those who smoke. OSA can also be the result of fatty deposits in the neck and throat, which act to further narrow the air passageway.

Complex, or Mixed, Sleep Apnea

This third form of sleep apnea is really just a combination of the other two, hence the "mixed" designation. There is local obstruction combined with a central (brain-based) disorder. Sort of like when traffic comes to a halt on the highway just before the tollbooths because of an accident in the left lane compounded by an electrical malfunction in some of the automated lanes. Because of its nature, complex sleep apnea must be treated with both kinds of interventions mentioned above.

WHAT PUTS THE ROAR IN SNORE?

A whopping 40 percent of all adults snore—so much for "Silent Night." Men make much more of this noise than women do—that is, until menopause comes on the scene. Then the ladies begin to join the nocturnal chorus in increasing numbers. There are five primary reasons that cause a person to join this nighttime jamboree.

1. *Obesity:* 70 percent of adults with sleep apnea have a body

mass index (BMI) in the obese category, which equals a BMI value of 30 or higher.*

2. *Decreased muscle tone:* Muscles that support the soft portion of your palate and your tongue begin to weaken, causing a structural collapse when you lie down and inhale.

3. *Abnormalities in your anatomy:* Physical obstruction from parts of your own body can partially block your airways. This can include a deviated septum (the cartilage separating your nostrils) or enlarged tonsils or adenoids, or an enlarged uvula.

4. *Nasal congestion:* When you and I lie down at night, the blood that gravity has drawn away from your sinuses because of your upright posture returns to the head, engorging the mucous membranes that line the sinus passages. Congestion can be made worse by colds, sinus infections, allergies, or chronic use of over-the-counter nasal sprays.

5. *Muscle-relaxing substances:* These include but are not limited to alcohol, tranquilizers, sleeping pills, and muscle-relaxant medications taken for pain relief.

Diagnosing Sleep Apnea

These days sleep apnea is a hot topic in the medical world and in the media. More and more laypeople are becoming aware of this potentially deadly disorder, and they are seeking answers and help from their doctors. (Hallelujah!) In response, sleep centers are popping up all across the county. During an appointment at a sleep center, after an initial exam, a patient will likely be scheduled for a sleep study (if the evaluating physician believes strongly the patient will prove to have sleep apnea). Here is a precaution: Make sure the

---

* See my website at www.lisamorrone.com/index.php/free-resources/bmi-calculator/ to determine your BMI.

doctor you have chosen to visit is board-certified in sleep medicine by the American Academy of Sleep Medicine. This way you know you have an expert on your case.

A sleep study, or *polysomnography*, is performed in a sleep laboratory. The patient lies down on the bed and is wired up from head to toe for an evening of monitoring and measuring. Then the patient is left to fall asleep—likely a bit difficult at first, but most everyone eventually does—at least long enough to record enough of the needed evidence. A complete polysomnography includes the following monitoring devices, measurements, and recordings:[4]

- an *electroencephalogram* (EEG), which monitors brain waves (sleep-stage information, seizure activity)

- an *electro-oculogram* (EOG), which monitors eye movements (sleep-stage information)

- an *electromyogram* (EMG), which monitors skeletal muscle activity (sleep-stage information, limb movement disorders)

- measurement of oral and nasal airflow

- *oximetry*, which measures blood-oxygen levels

- *measurement of chest and abdominal movement* (can distinguish between CSA and OSA)

- an *audio recording* of the loudness of snoring (for a little convincing, maybe?)

- and finally, *video monitoring*

The copious amount of data generated during this study is then analyzed by a board-certified sleep specialist (usually an otolaryngologist—an ENT—or a neurologist). Of particular interest is how many times the test subject has experienced a critical drop in airflow to their lungs. This number is then divided by the number of hours the person has been asleep. The result provides the average number of critical airflow dips per hour the patient has experienced, which serves as the basis for diagnosing the degree of apnea (see figure 7.1).

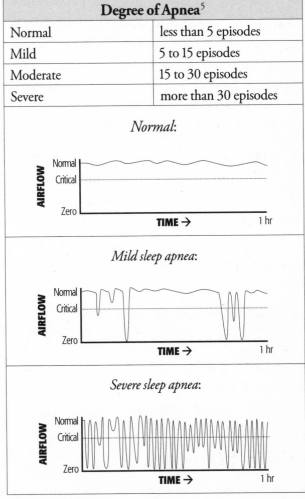

Degree of Apnea[5]	
Normal	less than 5 episodes
Mild	5 to 15 episodes
Moderate	15 to 30 episodes
Severe	more than 30 episodes

FIGURE 7.1

Once a diagnosis has been made (OSA, CSA, or mixed), and the severity has been determined (mild, moderate, or severe), the sleep specialist can begin to make recommendations. We will discuss these case-specific options and interventions as we move through the remainder of this chapter.

How Does Central Sleep Apnea Occur?

The brain-driven form of sleep apnea has often been years in the making. By that I mean it's typically the result of cardiovascular disease and is especially correlated with *atrial fibrillation* (A-fib) and *congestive heart failure. Brain tumors* and "brain attacks" (*strokes*) can also be initiators of CSA. Two other common risk factors, over which you have no control, are being part of the *male* population, and being *over the age of 65*. But like I said, no changing those two.

A sleep study can effectively distinguish between OSA and CSA because in OSA, the person's diaphragm and other muscles of respiration are actively contracting—trying to draw in a breath (against a local obstruction). In CSA, the breathing muscles are quiescent, or inactive—they haven't received the "Breathe now!" order from the commander-in-chief above.

The Top Eight Risk Factors for Obstructive Sleep Apnea

Since the majority of people with sleep apnea are diagnosed with OSA, the bulk of this chapter's discussion will focus there, with brief asides about CSA along the way. Sleep researchers have discovered that there are eight factors that significantly increase your risk of having sleep apnea. The encouraging thing here is, you have the power to change four of these eight. This means you could potentially reverse your sleep apnea condition without much medical intervention. That said, I do recommend you follow the advice of your sleep specialist.

Factors Under Your Control

1. *Overweight.* Excessive weight deposits fat throughout your body, including around your upper airway. This narrows your "breathe-way."

2. *Large neck circumference: more than 17 inches for men, and more than 16 inches for women.* Again, a thickened neck can narrow your internal airway passage. And necks tend to grow as bellies do, as we all know.

3. *Use of alcohol, sedatives, or tranquilizers.* Each of these substances acts to relax the muscles that surround the throat, leading to the collapse of structures into the airway. So steer clear of them at bedtime.

4. *Smoking.* By smoking—whether it is regular cigarettes or an evening cigar—you increase your risk of sleep apnea threefold. Nicotine, which is a chemical irritant, causes regional inflammation in your nasal passages, thickens your mucus secretions, and enlarges your adenoids. Yet another compelling reason to quit...

Factors Not Under Your Control

5. *Enlarged tonsils or adenoids.* Anything that is enlarged in the neighborhood of the throat will encroach upon the airway. Although you probably did not have a hand in creating this risk factor, you can take advantage of surgical treatment to reduce it. (As noted earlier, enlarged adenoids, which are troublesome in children under 12, are not likely to be an issue in the adult population, except among smokers.)

6. *Being male.* Your Y-chromosome has put you at risk, my male friend. So sorry...

7. *Being over 65 years of age.* As you and I age, the tone in our body's muscles begins to decline. This loss of tone weakens the support within the throat, allowing the soft palate, tonsils, adenoids, and tongue to flop into the upper airway. This is why the risk of getting sleep apnea is two to three times greater after you turn 65.

8. *A family history of sleep apnea.* Genetic factors associated with craniofacial structure, body fat distribution, and neural control of the upper airway muscles influence development of OSA.[6]

THE HOME SLEEP STUDY

The runner-up to the in-lab sleep study, in terms of accuracy of diagnosis and therefore treatment intervention, is the kind you can undergo at home. This is typically the next-best choice for people who don't have access to a sleep laboratory where they live, have been told the wait to be evaluated is beyond four months, have medical-insurance plans that simply won't cover the expense, or are extremely hesitant to sleep overnight in a "lab" (actually, a hospital-type room).

Now, not all devices for home sleep studies are the same. Those that include the ability to test for muscle tone and sleep position are best. That way you will get a more accurate assessment of your time asleep (since the severity of sleep apnea is measured by the number of apnea episodes per sleep time) and how your sleep position alters your airflow (for example, if you have very few episodes when asleep on your side but many when you are on your back, you may just need a position fix, not a positive airway pressure machine!).

Finally, if you go the route of a home study, it is imperative not only that your findings be analyzed by a sleep expert, but that you meet to discuss your results and subsequent treatment options with a board-certified sleep specialist. Anything less just won't do.

Why You Must Get Your Sleep Apnea Under Control

In 2008, a study was published in the scientific journal *Sleep* that confirmed the danger of untreated sleep apnea. Researchers followed a group of 380 adults, both men and women, who had been placed in three diagnostic groups: *severe sleep apnea, mild-to-moderate sleep apnea,* and *apnea-free.* After a period of 14 years researchers found that 33 percent of those subjects with severe sleep apnea had died, compared with only 7.7 percent of those without this condition.[7]

In another important study ("The Wisconsin Sleep Cohort") researchers followed 1522 adults, ages 30 to 60, over a period of 18 years. They found that those with sleep apnea at the start of the study were *two to three times* more likely to die from any cause when compared to those who did not have sleep apnea.[8] And here's yet another study, which found that 45 percent of participants who neglected to treat their moderate-to-severe sleep apnea suffered a significant cardiovascular event (heart attack or stroke) within the next 10 to 12 years![9]

If you value your time on this earth and the quality of health you have while you are here, there is almost nothing more important for you to do than to start a sleep investigation and then follow through with the recommendations of your sleep expert. Good nights equal a long life.

Treatment for Central Sleep Apnea

The initial course of action when attempting to minimize or correct the rarer problem of central sleep apnea, which is caused by a malfunction of the central nervous system, is to address the underlying medical problem. As noted, usually this is a cardiovascular issue, most typically *atrial fibrillation* or *congestive heart failure.* That said, it is often necessary to manage CSA with the use of some type of positive airway pressure machine (which will be more completely described in the section about treatment for obstructive sleep apnea).

Treatment for Obstructive Sleep Apnea

If you are diagnosed with sleep apnea, you can markedly improve your health and significantly perk up your energy level by employing the following treatment protocol.

Your Role

One of the most important things you can do to resolve or improve sleep apnea is to *lose weight*. This cannot be stressed enough. As noted earlier, being overweight leads to a fatty neck, which narrows your throat and obstructs your airway. It also places an extreme amount of pressure on your chest wall, which further narrows your airway because of the tugging effect all that belly fat has on your trachea (windpipe). The wonderful fact is that your weight-loss efforts will be enhanced once treatment of your sleep apnea has begun. This is because restored oxygen to your brain puts your body in a better metabolic state and your mind in a more motivated state. Significant weight loss will, hopefully, make your need for medical intervention a short-lived necessity.

Dr. Lee Shangold, the board-certified sleep specialist I mentioned earlier, has painstakingly graphed the results of over 1100 of his patients' sleep studies. Without exception, he found a direct correlation between a patient's BMI (Body Mass Index) and their *RDI* (Respiratory Disturbance Index, a similar, but even more sensitive measure than the earlier-defined AHI—the number of times your airflow drops below a critical level). Pound for pound, the heavier his patients were, the more they struggled to breathe, and the more severe their sleep apnea was. No wonder that study after study finds that the more weight a person with sleep apnea loses, the fewer apnea episodes they have per hour.* A mere 10 percent loss in body weight can cut your apnea events in half![10]

Another change, which is easy enough to make, is to alter your sleeping position. If you regularly sleep on your back, switch to sleeping on your side. This will help keep your tongue and soft palate out of the back of your throat. There are bed shirts (pajamas) that are designed with a foam wedge in the back. When you try to roll onto your back, the wedge guides you back onto your side. Just

---

* If you need help shedding some stubborn weight, you can find a very effective method in my books *Get Healthy, for Heaven's Sake* and *Overcoming Overeating*.

do an Internet search on "sleep apnea shirt" and follow the links. There are also U-shaped pillows that provide back and front support (two "walls," if you will) to help a person remain on their side throughout the night.

It is also critical that you avoid any substance that makes your tongue or soft palate any floppier than it already is. This means no alcohol consumption within three hours prior to sleep, and saying "no" to tranquilizers and sleeping pills. (It's funny that those sleeping pills can actually work against good sleep, isn't it? I'll bet that's not on the label!)

The final thing that can help to improve your oxygen intake at night is use products such as Breathe Right Strips and saline nasal spray. These aids will help to improve the airflow through your nasal passages. The more air you can take into your lungs, the more oxygen you make available to your brain. This way the commander-in-chief will quit waking you up all night to ask for more.

Seeking Medical Assistance

There are a number of medical interventions available that can aid in clearing the anatomical blockages that cause OSA. One noninvasive way to prevent your tongue from falling back into your throat at night is to get an *oral appliance*—a fitted bite plate or the acrylic tooth clip, NTI (Nociceptive Trigeminal Inhibition—see www.NTI-TSS.com). Both will guide your lower teeth and jaw to move forward, which in turn causes your tongue—which is attached to your jaw—to move forward as well, opening up your airway when you lie down.

The best candidates for successful treatment with an oral appliance meet the following criteria: 1) they have mild to moderate sleep apnea; 2) their apnea episodes occur much more often when they are lying on their backs rather than on their sides; and 3) their BMI (body mass index) is less than 30 (they are not obese).*

---

* For free resources, including a BMI calculator, see my website at www.lisamorrone.com/index.php/
free-resources.

The next mode of treatment requires surgery, which is performed primarily to improve the effectiveness of a positive airway pressure machine. If you are diagnosed with what is called *touching tonsils*, you will be advised to have those airway blockers removed as soon as possible. Other surgical procedures may be warranted if you are found to have additional fleshy obstructions. Greatly enlarged adenoids or an unduly fleshy uvula can be removed or downsized. And if you are unable to move air through your nose because of a deviated septum, rhinoplasty (an internal nose job) is another option. On rare occasions, palatal implant surgery, designed to structurally shore up a floppy soft palate, is advisable. But that would be a drastic procedure.

Usually sleep doctors do not go the surgical route (with the exception of removing touching tonsils). They tend to use an oral appliance and weight loss for mild OSA sufferers, and the CPAP (or *pneumatic stenting*) machine along with recommended weight loss for moderate-to-severe OSA patients.

Medical intervention via CPAP. Hands down, the most commonly prescribed medical intervention for sleep-apnea sufferers is the CPAP machine. It is used primarily for treatment of those with moderate-to-severe obstructive sleep apnea, though it is often used for central sleep apnea as well. The treatment it provides is revolutionary, truly lifesaving and life-enhancing.

As far as medical interventions go, the CPAP machine is relatively new to the market. Yet in the 30 years it has been in existence, sleep apnea has finally met its match. Basically the CPAP machine works to keep your airway propped open by maintaining a certain pressure blown into your nose, mouth, or both. The original pneumatic stent (*air splint*) machines provide an adjustable, consistent amount of pushed (or positive) air while you are inhaling *and* exhaling. Some patients find it troublesome to exhale against a stream of air of any force, and some people need so much positive air pressure to maintain a clear airway that they simply can't breathe out against it.

UNMASKING THE MYSTERY
OF POSITIVE AIRWAY PRESSURE DEVICES

Every machine used for the treatment of sleep apnea must have what is referred to as an *interface*. This is a fancy term for mask. It is how the device is able to effectively deliver the air you need without having it escape via an unwanted route.

Traditionally the mask was a hard plastic piece that was fitted over the nose and mouth or just the nose, and it was held in place by elastic strapping. Today there are a couple of other options. The first are nasal pillows. This interface can be worn by those who do not have nasal obstructions, and who regularly breathe through their nose while they sleep. Basically it is a set of nose plugs with air tubes running through them.

The second nontraditional option available is what is called "no mask." Sound promising? Well, more accurately it should be called "no straps." It consists only of a mouthpiece that is fitted to your bite to hold it in place and two small tubes that deliver the air pressure into your nostrils. This is a wonderful option if all those head straps are deterring you from beginning treatment. So if the thought of having something covering your nose and mouth has you feeling claustrophobic, one of these alternatives may be right for you.

For either of these two situations, the newer *BiPAP*, or Bi-level Positive Airway Pressure, produces a dual level of air pressure—more during the inhalation and less during exhalation. It does this by sensing when a patient has begun to exhale, and then reducing its blowing pressure by a prescribed increment. This dual airflow feature has greatly improved patient comfort and compliance levels.

Another more advanced model, the *auto-titrating CPAP*, or more simply the *APAP*, machine has the ability to sense just how much pressure is needed to maintain an open airway and deliver exactly what is needed. Because it is more specialized, it is of course more expensive. Often this machine is used for home sleep studies. That noted, this device is a great match for those patients who need a bit of air splinting when they are in non-REM sleep but a whole lot more when they are in REM sleep, or for those who have significantly different stenting needs based upon their position (side-lying or back-lying).

Finally, another intelligent device that has been recently introduced is the *adaptive servo-ventilator*, or *ASV*. This machine, similarly to the APAP, can sense when you are having difficulty breathing and when you are not. When you need help with airway support, it's there; when you don't, it backs off and lets you take over the task of breathing. It acts much like a ventilator you'd see in a hospital, minus the endotracheal tube. It has been shown to reduce the work of breathing by 50 percent. This device is typically reserved for the CSA population.

If you are still thinking, *Not me—I could never get used to sleeping with a mask on my face and a machine "breathing" alongside my bed*, just take a moment to read the testimonials of your once oxygen-deprived fellow sufferers. They may convince you to go ahead and investigate this medical intervention.

CPAP "Survivor" Stories

Terry

Many years ago I was told that I snored loudly and even "sputtered" in my sleep. Truthfully, I regularly felt tired when I awoke—like I could never get enough sleep. When I finally talked with my doctor about this issue, he first performed a test which monitored my oxygen level during one night's sleep. This preliminary test revealed that my oxygen dipped dangerously low—so low that he immediately referred me to a sleep specialist.

That very week I had a traditional sleep study done, and the results were not good. On average I had stopped and restarted breathing more than 30 times an hour! That rate placed me in the severe apnea category. I was given a CPAP machine and sent home to get used to it.

I must say the transition of sleeping with the CPAP was an easy one for me. I haven't missed a night since I began using it. I guess I was so motivated because I felt immediate positive results. Each morning I wake feeling much less tired, my overall health has improved, and I find that I concentrate much better throughout my day. So remarkable is the change between my "before" and "after" that I never fail to have it with me even on business trips and vacation.

Carole

Ever since I was a little girl I have been falling asleep in the most unusual places…during snack time at school, at the kitchen table, at the movies, in church services, while on hold on the telephone, while reading, while standing, as a passenger on every car ride—and each day, like clockwork, at 3 p.m. I even fell asleep once while pedaling an exercise bike! Many days, when I was driving, I would have to pull my car over to the side of the road to nap just so I could make it home alive.

I began to believe that my constant tiredness must be my own fault. I was obviously not getting enough rest at night. But truthfully, no matter what time I went to bed I woke up weary, wishing the day would fly by so I could get back under the covers. I began to question my doctors regarding a possible cause for my chronic exhaustion. The first physician I asked said it was a side effect of the medicine I was taking for my depression. My primary doctor said that I had a vitamin D deficiency. Another said it could be the onset of menopause (having lasted since I was a little girl?). None of the medical doctors I visited asked me any additional questions about my condition, and when they seemed unconcerned, I just left the issue alone.

Sometime later my family and I took a cruise together. One morning, my daughter said, "You know, Mom, you sound like you are going to die at night. You stop breathing all the time. I find myself anxiously waiting for you to start breathing again. And…you snore." Honestly I was more mortified by the thought of me, a lady, snoring! When we came back home I decided it was time I made an appointment for a sleep study.

To my horror, my sleep study found that I was waking up between 15 and 30 times in any given hour—no wonder I woke up tired every morning! I was diagnosed with both central and obstructive sleep apnea. My sleep specialist prescribed a BiPAP machine, and I was fitted with a mask.

It took me about three months to work up to using the BiPAP for the whole night—the machine's noise and the wearing of the mask took some getting used to. Now I use it every single night because with it, I am a new woman— one who wakes up rested and can stay awake all day. Once, when I went away with a friend, I left my machine home only out of fear of embarrassment. What a mistake! I woke up exhausted and irritable.

In hindsight I wish I had known a couple of things. First, there are different types of masks available, and choosing the right one should not be rushed. Secondly, I wasn't informed that there were monthly insurance co-pays I would be responsible for—and in my case they were a bit hefty. Though I must admit, the change to my life has been so remarkable that I would pay twice what I do now.

But now let me tell you the best part of using the BiPAP— yes, even better than waking up refreshed. The depression I battled for years has finally subsided. You see, the medication that I had been taking was only partially effective. A few months after I began treatment for my sleep apnea, my "depression fog" lifted. I feel better than I have in years!

Casey

For years, I would feel very tired (more like sluggish) during the day, and I always felt like I was out of breath. My husband had complained many times that he could not get a good night's sleep because I was snoring too loudly. He once taped me and replayed the tape for me in the morning. I was horrified to find out that the "horrible sound" was coming from me!

Well, it finally came to a head when he sat up in bed one night, almost on the verge of tears, telling me I *must* do something about my snoring. At that point, I decided to visit an ENT, who observed that I had a deviated septum and that I was a good candidate for a sleep study.

Later that week, I had my sleep study. The following day, the doctor's office called me to say that my results put me in the same category as a 500-pound male! I had stopped breathing 101 times an hour, and my heart rate had dropped below 60. I was told that people have been known to die in their sleep from such a severe form of sleep apnea, and they stressed the urgency of my getting on a CPAP unit immediately—which I did.

Surprisingly, it only took about two or three days for me to get used to sleeping with it. I use my CPAP unit seven nights a week, and I even bring it on vacation. It's been nearly four years since I began using it, and it has become something I cannot do without. Each morning I wake up feeling well rested, and I am no longer out of breath during the day. (I have to say, I think it even reduced the swelling around my eyes!)

Chapter 8

Restless Legs Syndrome

What to Do When Your Legs Won't Sleep

There are so many things in life that can work against a good night's sleep. We began the self-help portion of this book talking about external factors such as bedtime routines, dietary influences, and bedroom environments. From there we turned our attention to some of the most-often-encountered internal factors—beginning with bladder-control issues. Next we addressed two very common sleep problems: physical pain and obstructive sleep apnea, both of which are responsible for waking people during the night, whether they know it (for example, pain) or not (for example, sleep apnea).

That brings us to the next sleep deterrent: *restless legs*. Personally I believe this problem should be spelled this way—*rest-less* legs—because if you suffer from this condition, that about sums up their effect on your sleep. Your legs move more, so you rest less.

The first time I heard about restless legs syndrome, Nancy Sinatra's hit 1960s song, "These Boots Are Made for Walkin'," popped into my head. That was the soundtrack my mind chose for a scene in which feet were on the move involuntarily. While the song's lyrics might conjure up a humorous image, for the people who must live with this limb-movement disorder, having "rest-less legs" is no laughing matter.

A Syndrome That's Got Legs

In 1944, the condition originally called *irritable legs* was described by Dr. Karl Ekbom, a physician. A year later, he renamed it *restless legs syndrome*, or RLS. To date that name has stuck, despite the growing opinion among sufferers, who believe it makes their condition sound simply bothersome rather than altogether maddening and life-altering.

Restless legs syndrome is a neurologic, brain-driven movement disorder that prompts the afflicted person to keep their legs in motion to temporarily lessen or eliminate aggravating leg sensations. Typically, these strange sensations kick into gear by the early evening, just as their owner is attempting to settle down from the day's activity. Though they can be ignored for a bit, the annoyance level will build until the person is compelled to move their legs. Try sleeping with all that motion going on!

This dreadful syndrome prevents millions of people from falling asleep every night. Unlike the overactive bladder, which wakes someone periodically from a sound sleep, RLS is a condition that afflicts a person when they are awake—though desperately trying not to be.

The symptoms are most pronounced between the hours of 11 p.m. to 3 a.m.—ruining some of the best sleep a night has to offer. The troubling sensations typically (and thankfully) subside by early morning so the RLS sufferer can finally get a few hours of much-needed rest. Even so, there is still a huge load of sleep debt left to carry around. It comes as no surprise that people with RLS feel tired, irritable, and anxious, especially as evening approaches.

While the precise cause of restless legs syndrome is still unknown, what scientists have discovered is that RLS has something to do with one of the brain's neurotransmitters, *dopamine*. Dopamine deficiency has long been understood to be the underlying cause of Parkinson's disease, another neurologically driven movement disorder characterized by resting tremors, stiffened muscles, and a shuffling gait. Thankfully, people with RLS have no greater risk of developing Parkinson's disease than those without it.[1]

SENSATIONS AND SYMPTOMS

Most people who suffer with RLS describe an annoying sensation felt deep within their legs. (Although some people don't specify a particular sensation. All they know is, they've gotta move!) The intensity of this sensation builds over time until there is no other choice but to move the affected limbs to get some relief. Below you'll find a list of attempts to describe these symptoms. Can you find yours among them?

crawling	tense
tingling	uncomfortable
cramping	itchy
creeping	tugging
pulling	gnawing
painful	aching
electric	burning

Do You Have the URGE to Move?

To see if your problem fits the bill for RLS, the National Institutes of Health and the International Restless Legs Syndrome Study Group (yes, there is such an organization) have joined forces to bring you four clear-cut must-haves to indicate this diagnosis. They are based on the acronym URGE:

Uncontrollable need to move your legs. Deep within the legs is a sensation that refuses to be ignored. Its intensity grows until moving your limbs becomes an urgent matter—much like scratching at an inflamed mosquito bite. While you can hold off this response for a while, in the end your legs will win out and you absolutely must move them. This deep-sourced irritation sets RLS apart from other sensation-driven disorders, which are instead described as being at the surface level or skin-deep. (*Note*: While most people report the discomfort in their legs, some also experience similar complaints in their arms, trunk, or face.)

Rest-induced. Without exception, RLS symptoms worsen during periods of mental or physical inactivity, such as when a person is seated or lying down. Many people who do not have nighttime symptoms report getting these leg disturbances during a long flight or while watching a very long movie. My husband typically experiences this during flights to or from Europe or when flying coast-to-coast in the U.S. It's one reason he always books an aisle seat—that and his extra-long legs.

Most disturbing for the RLS sufferer is the fact that the longer the resting period, the more pronounced the symptoms become. Mentally stimulating activities such as playing video games, watching television, or reading may help prevent the onset of symptoms (at least in the early stage of the disorder). While that may help the early evening symptoms, what good is it when you are trying to fall asleep?

Gets better with activity. This third must-have characteristic is obvious to those who suffer with RLS. When their legs build up with noxious tension, they instinctively know that moving their limbs will make them feel better. As mentioned above, symptom relief can be achieved by engaging in some sort of mentally stimulating activity. My husband noticed that as long as he continued to watch TV or work on his laptop during a flight, his legs felt fine. As soon as he closed his eyes to sleep, his legs would act up and he'd feel compelled to jump up into the aisle. When RLS first appears, activity typically brings complete or nearly complete relief. Yet as the years go on, physical movement and distracting mental activity seem to become less effective and, sadly, only partial symptom relief is achieved.

Evening accentuation. The severity of RLS symptoms follows the body's circadian rhythm. They tend to increase as the evening arrives and then reach their peak, as noted earlier, between 11 p.m. and 3 a.m., making it difficult, if not impossible, to get a restful night's sleep.

RANKING YOUR RESTLESSNESS[2]

Severity	Time of day when symptoms begin (more than 50 percent of the time)
Mild	Bedtime
Moderate	Evening (starting after 6 p.m.)
Severe	Afternoon (after 12 p.m.)
Very severe	Morning (before noon)

Who Suffers from RLS?

While you may never have heard of RLS until this chapter, restless legs syndrome is quite common. It afflicts about 10 percent of the adult population in the U.S. Of those, about one-third, or 3 percent of the U.S. population, have symptoms severe enough to require medical intervention.[3] (We will discuss what that looks like below.)

Surprisingly, unlike Parkinson's disease, which affects more men than women, the incidence of RLS is about twice as high in females as in males.[4] Its incidence also increases as you get older, especially older than 50. And once RLS begins, while there may be periods of reprieve, it tends to pick up speed. As the years progress, an affected person will likely find that their symptoms will 1) begin earlier in the day, 2) increase in intensity, and 3) resolve less completely in response to moving their limbs.

DO BUSY LEGS RUN IN THE FAMILY?

Studies have found a family history of RLS in more than 50 percent of people who suffer from it. Furthermore, when compared with those who are not affected, a person with RLS is three to six times more likely to have a positive family history of it.[5]

Recently, genetic researchers in Germany have identified underlying gene mutations in individuals who begin experiencing symptoms before the age of 30. Because of their unusual gene pool, those with early-onset RLS have a 50 percent chance of passing this genetic mutation down to their children. Probably not the inheritance they were hoping to leave their kids!

Are Your Legs Under the Influence?

For the majority with RLS, an underlying medical problem does not exist. However, in rare instances, RLS has been shown to accompany other medical conditions. By directly addressing these co-existing health issues you may be able to put an end to this tormenting nocturnal disorder.[6] Let's take a brief look at the possible negative influences your legs may be under.

Peripheral neuropathy. Damaged nerve endings—most frequently in the hands and feet—are often the product of poorly regulated blood sugar (diabetes) or chronic alcoholism. Sensation changes can vary from numbness or tingling to outright pain. Peripheral neuropathy can also result from chemotherapy treatment or from disc damage or a pinched spinal nerve. In these cases, the sensation changes can present themselves anywhere along the arm or leg. Medications are available today that act directly on these irritated nerve endings, bringing some relief of the noxious, possibly RLS-provoking, symptoms.

Iron deficiency. You don't need to have full-blown anemia to cause or increase RLS symptoms. Iron deficiency can result from repeated stomach or rectal bleeding associated with ulcers or hemorrhoids. Even heavy menstrual periods or repeated blood donation (more than six times per year) can drop your iron levels to an unhealthy level. A simple blood test can determine a deficiency, which can be rectified with either an iron supplement or by eating iron-rich foods such as spinach, egg yolks, or red meat.

Kidney failure. When your kidneys fail to function properly, iron stores in your blood can decrease. This leads to iron deficiency and eventually to full-blown anemia. This, along with other changes in body chemistry from malfunctioning kidneys, may cause or worsen RLS. Simple blood and urine tests can give your physician a good idea as to how well your kidneys are functioning.

Other culprits. While pregnancy is a wonderful event in so many ways, during the third trimester the "host body" is usually not feeling so chipper. This is when RLS can begin to occur. Thankfully, the condition will typically fade from existence within four weeks after delivery.[7] Alcohol use and sleep deprivation (before the onset of RLS) are two other factors that may aggravate or trigger the symptoms in some individuals.[8] Finally, some over-the-counter and prescription "anti" medications have been shown to stimulate RLS. These include antinausea, antipsychotic, antidepressant, and antihistamine drugs. (Not all "anti" meds will have this unwelcomed effect. Always check with your doctor or pharmacist for drug side-effect information.)

TIRED OF BEING KICKED AROUND

Busy legs make bad bed partners. Over the years I have spoken with many people who have had to banish their "kicking" partner from their bed or have chosen to evacuate the bedroom themselves in search of a less stimulating sleeping arrangement.

If you and your legs are sleeping alone when you'd prefer to be sleeping with your bed buddy, realize it's not *you* your partner wants to get away from—it's those busy legs of yours. Don't allow those overactive limbs to come between the two of you. I hope that by using the information from this chapter you will finally be able to hush those limbs. Then I'm sure you'll be welcomed back—legs and all!

Coaxing Your Legs to Settle Down

The first go-to for your health issues should not be medication. Medicines, especially those used to treat RLS, can come with unwanted strings attached. (More on this topic in just a bit.) That said, there are lifestyle changes that have been shown to impact restless legs for the better. You are better off attempting to combat your symptoms on your own, at least before they become unmanageable, using these methods:

- *Reduce caffeine.* If you drink more than two cups of caffeinated beverages each day, it's time to reel that in, my friend. That way there will be less caffeine coursing through your body to hype up your legs.

- *Say goodbye to cigarettes and alcohol.* Beyond the other obvious health benefits, people with RLS report improvement in their symptoms when these bad boys are apprehended and run out of town.

- *Lose weight.* Shedding 10 percent of your body weight is a great goal to begin with when you're attempting to positively influence your RLS symptoms. Though it is uncertain as to how being overweight influences your brain's dopamine processing, it has been adequately demonstrated that weight loss equals symptom loss. (Need help battling your bulge? Pick up my book *Overcoming Overeating*.)

- *Exercise...but only in moderation.* Your exercise routine should include aerobic activity and stretching for the large muscle groups in the legs (calves, quadriceps, and hamstrings). Strenuous exercise, on the other hand, can actually have the opposite effect, worsening your restless legs' symptoms—so participate at your own risk.

- *Take vitamin supplements.* Have your doctor check your blood to see if you are low in iron, vitamin B, folic acid, or magnesium. If so, add any deficient elements back to your diet in the form of nutrient-dense food or supplements and see if you can get your RLS to settle down.

- *Find a stress-buster.* Increased emotional stress also plays a role in exacerbating the symptoms of RLS. Take a swim, go dancing, play a game, garden, pray, sing—whatever you find enjoyable. Make sure you allow time to power down each day in some way so you avoid taking all that stress to bed with you at night.

- *Follow a consistent sleep schedule.* Since fatigue can heighten symptoms, set your sights on a 7- to 8-hour sleep period. Unwind by taking a warm bath before climbing into bed, and then settle into a good read before dozing off.

Medications That Make a Difference

If you have put into practice all you've learned in this book and still can't get your legs to settle down for the night, then medication is your last frontier. To date, two medicines have been approved by the FDA specifically for the treatment of RLS: Mirapex (pramipexole) and Requip (ropinirole).[9] Both of these are dopamine-related medications similar to the ones used for the treatment of Parkinson's disease. Other off-label meds (approved for use in other conditions, but found to be effective with RLS) include a number of anticonvulsant, anti-anxiety, and pain-reliever varieties.[10] Under the direction of your physician, you can begin to explore the possibilities of pharmaceuticals.

GOING FROM BAD TO WORSE

If you absolutely can't get your legs to sleep, it's likely you'll turn to prescription medicine—I know I would. The only problem with long-term use of these dopamine-based drugs is that a condition known as *augmentation* may begin. The word *augment* means to enhance, or expand—and that is just what can occur with your symptoms. Over time, some people report that not only do their RLS symptoms start to show up earlier in the day (bad), but the symptoms themselves become more intense (worse), and even begin to take up more real estate in their body (much worse). See why I was cautious about using medicinal intervention out of the gate?

If you begin to experience signs of augmentation, please tell your doctor as soon as possible. You may need to change the way you take your medicine or switch to a different medicine or combination of medicines.[11]

Double Trouble: RLS with Periodic Limb Movement

Unfortunately, more than 80 percent of people with RLS also experience a condition known as *periodic limb movement of sleep* (PLMS). Unlike RLS, whose associated leg movements take place when a person is awake, PLMS occurs while you are asleep. During sleep studies, PLMS incidences are found to occur one to four times per minute on average. Often these involuntary leg twitches or jerking movements go unnoticed by the one doing the kicking. (But not by the one who must dodge all the kicks—review the "Tired of Being Kicked Around" sidebar.) On occasion, though, some people will experience leg jerks strong enough to repeatedly wake themselves during the night, thoroughly disrupting their sleep.

This combination is most definitely tormenting—having to live with legs you are compelled to move while you're awake, compounded with the continuous leg motion that occurs once sleep does set in. The good news is that medications which bring relief to RLS sufferers have been shown to settle down PLMS symptoms as well. (If your periodic leg movements of sleep are present without any sign of RLS, they go by the name *periodic limb movement disorder*, or PLMD. If you are losing sleep because of PLMD, don't hesitate to visit your doctor. There may be a remedy for your situation.)

Regardless of the severity of your undesired leg movement, you have the power to do a lot to stack the odds in favor of a full night's sleep. Apply the suggested lifestyle changes first, and then use medications as your last resort. I wish you success in your quest to live at peace with your legs once again!

Chapter 9

Attack of the Busy Brain

Learn to Ease Your Mind and Calm Your Emotions

The other day my son, Adam, smiled sheepishly as he confessed to me, "Mom, I know this is going to sound weird for a teenager to say, but I've been so exhausted for the past six months—getting up early for school—that I actually get *excited* when I realize that my bedtime is approaching! Isn't that pitiful?" "No, Adam," I mused, "that is what it's like to be an adult. Welcome to my world!"

On evenings when you've had "too much day" I'm sure you begin to look forward to your bedtime with as much enthusiasm as my son does. *Thank goodness, the time is finally here...* Pajama-clad, you turn off the lights and slide in between the sheets. You roll to your side and snuggle in. Then you exhale...long and slow...and that's when you hear it. It begins faintly as a hushed voice muffled by the crinkling sound of your pillowcase. And then it builds...and now it's a full-blown chattering. Your brain has roared to life. And that voice—it's yours.

Ugh, not tonight.

Your body is beyond tired. You've had a full day and you anticipate another jam-packed day tomorrow. Would someone *please* tell your brain that it's time to power down? Doesn't it know that this is *its* time to rest as well?

I believe much of this problem has to do with how we've trained our minds. For those of you with "busy brains," discipline and redirection of your thought life is going to be the key to turning off your brain so you can rest. If children are raised without guidance or discipline, chances are they will begin to run amok as they grow older. The same holds true for the brain. You and I can take control of our thought life, redirect it, and even get it to give us a rest. It is indeed possible—even though at this point you may be having doubts.

Over the 40-some years of my life I have lost many a night to a busy brain. Truthfully, most of us who swim about in this stressful soup we call life will suffer a busy-brain attack from time to time—it simply comes with the territory. This chapter will be helpful for those of you who encounter the occasional attack, but it can be life-changing for those of you suffering from the chronic condition. You're the unfortunate person who's been struggling to fall asleep for years, maybe even for as long as you can remember. You are wound up like a top most of the time, and when you finally lie down at night, all your brain does is spin, spin, spin. Well, you are about to enter the "no-spin zone."

Today in Review

Why do our brains rewind and replay our day when we are trying to fall asleep? It seems the scenes that first project themselves on the back of our eyelids are those of all our unfinished business. The work presentation due on Friday that you've yet to begin, the piles of unwashed laundry, the doctor's appointment you keep forgetting to schedule. Then you move on to think about the parts of the day that didn't go as planned. Your car tire blew out on the way into work, one of your customers called with a complaint (which turned the rest of your day on its end), the dog left you a "present" on the carpet, your teenager lost his retainer…and on and on it goes.

This painful rehashing of your day only leaves you feeling unaccomplished and agitated. Both of these emotions trigger the release of adrenaline, which acts to speed up your body's heart and breathing rate. This ill-timed hormone release prepares your body for a fight-or-flight response rather than lulling you to sleep. It is the antithesis of melatonin's effect. Now who needs that?

A few years ago, I made a decision to rein in my brain at night. I defined new boundaries for my "day in review." Before I drifted off to sleep, I determined I would only think about what made me smile that day, what I had accomplished, and how God had helped me to be a blessing to someone else. In a word, I limited my review to what had made that day a good one. If another thought began to form that did not meet my criteria, I immediately stopped that reflection in its tracks and promptly replaced it with something pleasant. After a few times of getting its toes stepped on, my brain, with its free-range thoughts, learned its lesson and stayed within my new parameters.

Press Pause

If our brains were as easy to direct as our television's remote control, we could simply press "pause" before we slid into bed. But we are man (or woman), not machine. Now and then a thought pops into my head while I am relaxing to sleep—an idea, or something I need to think about or remember for the next day. My brain is stuck on it for fear of forgetting it. Here is where a pad of paper and a pen come in very handy. For years I have kept these two items on my night table for times like this. I jot down that "must remember" thought or idea, and then I find I can get my brain to release its tenacious grip on it.

Ever wonder where the saying "Let me sleep on it" comes from? Some of you may have heard the scientific fact that our brains actually problem-solve and analyze information while we sleep. Therefore I have given my brain the full responsibility to do just that—without me having to be involved. Think about it—would you wash your car before taking it to the car wash? Why think through a situation and lose an hour of sleep if your brain can work on it for you *while* you sleep? Deliberately press "pause" on all those busy thoughts, allow your subconscious to work on them through the night, and you'll find you are better prepared to handle all the details of the next day.

WHATCHA THINKIN' ABOUT?

Comedian Jerry Seinfeld does a shtick where he asks the women in his audience if they would like to know what their men are thinking—*really* thinking—as they go about their day. He admits he's not even supposed to tell them, but if they would *really* like to know (and, of course, his female audience cheers him on), he will tell them.

And then comes a pregnant pause. Finally, Jerry blurts out the long-awaited answer: "Nothing—absolutely nothing! They're just walkin' around, lookin' around!"

Fast-Forward

We just spoke of learning to press the pause button—yet every day our world seems bent on continually hitting the fast-forward button for us. Our to-do lists far outlast our waking hours—even though we are flying through our days at breakneck speed. Lunch hours are squeezed into five minutes in front of our computers, and break times are limited to getting up and pouring yourself another cup of java. How can we expect to zoom though the day and then go from a hundred miles per hour to a complete stop in a matter of minutes?

When I was the captain of the track team in high school one of my responsibilities was to make sure the team had a sufficient cooldown before they headed back to the locker room. Runners in training never finish a hard workout and then just sit down. To unwind their muscles they jog at a slow pace, they stretch, and then they take a warm shower. A runner will also use this cooldown time to reflect on the training they have just completed. If these slowdown and reflection steps are skipped, the runner's body is at risk for injury and he will not be mentally prepared as well as he could be for his next practice or race.

Think of your day like that. Sprint if you must, but make sure you have the time to unwind your brain's thoughts before climbing into bed. Set aside time to reflect on your day—what you've learned, what you've accomplished, or what you'd still like to achieve. If you neglect to give your brain the free time to process your day *as it's in progress*, it will steal precious time from your night to accomplish this most needful task.

The Event Planner on Overdrive

Hello. My name is Lisa, and I'm a plan-a-holic.

As far back as I can remember I have tried to plan the future. At age ten, I recall carefully tracking the earnings I made from being a mother's helper, with the specific goal of purchasing my first stereo system. My father had said he would match my funds dollar for dollar, so I had my eyes on a new stereo with an AM-FM radio, a turntable, and an eight-track tape player. I had priced out the model I wanted and bit by bit, I moved toward my goal. Eventually the day arrived, and I brought that new stereo system home.

So how does someone like me (or you), a compulsive planner, refrain from planning out the next day's events while lying in bed? Here's what has been working for me: I make sure I have the next day's schedule thought through and written down somewhere before I get into bed. That way I am not tempted to detail out the upcoming day while my head is on my pillow.

And here is another attitude I take to bed with me that might work for some of you. It stems from my personal relationship with Jesus Christ. In my prayers I let God know that although I have planned my next day, He has full rights to mess with my schedule—for His glory. Because I have given God free rein, I don't have to lie there and fret about the possible disruptions that may occur in my tomorrow. I know that whatever happens, the Lord will cause all things to work together for good, because I love Him and I am called according to His purposes (see Romans 8:28).

All Wound Up and No Place to Go

If you find that you frequently lie in bed at night completely unable to calm your mind—and if you can feel your heart and pulse rate doing the cha-cha—you may need to discover an effective method to process the stressors in your life during the daytime. Think about this: All those thoughts racing through your head at night are actually present all day long; they're just not accounted for. You have busied yourself to the point of distraction. In the dark hours of the night, when there are no other diversions, your suppressed thoughts take center stage.

There are many positive ways to process your issues and de-stress yourself throughout the day. Why don't you try one of these on for size?

- *Journal*—process your emotions and thoughts through the written word

- *Pray*—lift up your concerns and requests to God

- *Exercise*—with regularity (just not too late in the evening)

- *Read fiction books*—entering a world other than your own can be calming

- *Take up a pleasurable hobby*—this balances out the unpleasant parts of your day

- *Take a hot shower or soak in a warm bath*—this will have an all-over soothing effect

- *Speak to a counselor, pastor, or dear friend*—someone who will offer sound advice

- *Socialize*—get out and about on a regular basis and you'll find your tension will ease as your rekindle and maintain people connections

The Blame Game—Target, *You*

Coulda, shoulda, woulda…you know the mantra. Mentally you beat yourself up while you're lying down. You second-guess yourself—actions, words, maybe even motives. What you have here is a routine attack of "It's all my fault"—something that's based less on reality and more on your own insecurities. Quit the negative, unwarranted self-analysis and offer yourself a generous portion of grace—I've heard there's a limitless supply. This way you can stop cutting into yourself at night and start sawing wood instead.

Other times, however, there's no question about it—you know you're at fault. You have wronged someone, been dishonest, acted badly. And now the memory of it all comes flooding back…just when you thought it was safe to turn out the lights. You may be wrestling with deep remorse as you lie there in bed shaming yourself night after night. So where do you go to get closure so you can get some rest?

The Magic Eraser for guilt, plain and simple, is forgiveness. It's the *only* thing that can permanently remove this stubborn stain from your life. Forgiveness comes in three forms, each with the ability to change guilt into peace. However, the precursor to receiving any type of forgiveness is a clear admission of guilt—confession, that is. You need to verbally take responsibility for what you did or the part you played, no finger-pointing allowed. You guilt is your own regardless of whether or not you had accomplices.

Form 1: Forgiveness from people. It may be that the person or people you have wronged may not want to forgive you. That is their issue. Whatever the outcome, your responsibility is to simply and humbly state your guilt (without backup explanation) and ask to be forgiven. The guilt-removing power of forgiveness comes from the act of honest confession and the request to be forgiven, *not* from having the other party accept your apology—though that always makes a better closure.

Form 2: Forgiveness from God. Those of you who live your life in a faith-based way realize that the second form of forgiveness is indispensable. You must ask God to forgive you. I believe that while we are fully capable of *hurting* others, we can only *sin* against our Creator. Therefore, if we are looking to resolve the guilt problem that keeps us up at night, we would do well to seek His pardon.

Form 3: Forgiveness from yourself. Finally, you and I must be willing—after following through with the first two forms of forgiveness—to forgive ourselves. And here is where many people get hung up. Some will hold onto something that was long ago pardoned by their Savior and even by the one who they wronged, thinking of it as a sort of penitence or punishment. These people (possibly you are one of them) cannot seem to shake their regret—and they revisit it most every night.

This practice is painful and unproductive—and thoroughly unnecessary. If you have sincerely asked for forgiveness from the one true Judge, Jesus Christ—who is ready, willing, and able to pardon the humble in heart—who are you to not offer forgiveness to yourself? By being unwilling to forgive yourself, you are placing your judgment above God's. As well-known Bible teacher Beth Moore likes to say, when we beat ourselves up with guilt over something God has already forgiven, He doesn't look down from heaven and say, "Oh, aren't you so humble?"—He says, "Aren't you faithless?" Choose to believe Him for what He has already done.

DON'T COUNT SHEEP—COUNT ON THE SHEPHERD

I never understood why we were told as children to count sheep when we were having trouble sleeping. Were we to count them in a herd, or one by one jumping over a fence? I wasn't even sure if sheep could jump.

I guess what our parents were saying is this: Try to bore yourself to sleep (as if lying on your back in a dark room with nothing else to do wasn't boring enough!). When that "sheepish approach" failed to produce sleep, I tried a different method that I discovered to be far more effective—prayer to the One who is called the Good Shepherd in the Bible.

Now stay with me here. I am not saying that prayer is boring. I am saying that when I direct my thoughts to prayer, my body and mind relax. Then I can easily drift off to sleep.

I will lie down and sleep in peace, for you alone,
O LORD, make me dwell in safety.[1]

Tomorrow's Forecast: Doom and Gloom

If what is unseen in your future seriously worries you, you are probably an accomplished pessimist—someone who reads doom and gloom into almost everything. Likely you keep yourself up, or wake yourself up, because your mind is racked with fear, worry, and anxiety. If fretful worrying or full-blown anxiety attacks had the ability to assist you in any way with the actual outcomes in your life, then I'd say, "Have at it!" But the reality is, these emotions are useless, and worse yet, harmful to marinate in.

Troublesome thoughts enter into everyone's mind from time to time. You get to decide, however, if those thoughts will be allowed to speak their piece, if they will be entertained and asked to stay on awhile, or if they will abruptly be shown the door. It really is that simple (though not always easy). The Bible says that we have the ability to take every thought captive, which means we have more power over our thoughts than they can have over us.[2] This is an important fact to remind yourself of in the dead of night when fear and worry stand over you, poised for attack. Myself, I make it a rule not to worry about something until I know there is something to be concerned about—and by that time worry (which is about the future) doesn't have a role to play. I can move straight into action when I know what I'm dealing with. The only thing I do about the future is pray…and plan, of course.

"And Now I Lay Me Down to Seethe…"

Been there, done that, bought the T-shirt. Anger and I go way back, all the way back to my upbringing in a dysfunctional home run by broken people. As I grew older, though, I began to realize I was using anger as a weapon. And when I grew older still, I discovered that the weapon I was wielding was actually damaging me more than those I directed it toward.

Had I paid more attention in my Sunday-school classes, I might have remembered God's directives regarding anger. Basically He has two things to say on the subject. First, don't let the sun go down on your anger,[3] or to put it another way, don't go to bed angry. And second, in your anger do not sin.[4]

Now I love stew—but not at night. Stewing in your anger always results in something tough to chew on, and it gets tougher the longer you let it simmer. Do yourself a favor and keep a short record of wrongs. Be quick to forgive. It doesn't mean that what was done to you is now acceptable; it simply allows you to be released from the bondage of unforgiveness.

And what about that second biblical directive? Is anger a wrong or sinful reaction? Absolutely not. Scripture specifies "*In* your anger, do not sin." Anger can be a righteous response (though not always—see my book *Overcoming Headaches and Migraines*, chapter 12). We must be careful to not get caught in sin's trap because of our anger. When we handle our anger in an unhealthy way, we become unhealthy—beginning with the loss of sleep we can suffer.

As an adult, when I finally was able to understand the purpose of obeying those two directives, I found such freedom—which translated into consistently restful sleep. These days, whenever someone asks me if it was difficult to become a Christian because of all the things I had to give up, I always answer, "Yes, I did have to give up many things—anger, bitterness, fear…" God knew that great peace comes from living in harmony with others (as far as it depends on us) and being at peace with Him. That is why He gave us His take on the whole anger-management thing. Peace with Him is the result of a life characterized by confessed wrongdoing along with the goal to do what is right—according to His holy Word. Now that's something you can sleep on!

A busy brain can and will attack the best of us from time to time. The key is learning how not to let our minds run away with our sleep night after night. I truly hope that you will take this chapter to heart. It is always helpful and profitable to process your emotions during the day so you can devote your full night to sleep.

Chapter 10

"Just Take a Pill..."

Supplements and Medications—Are They Really Worth It?

S ometimes when you've done your best and tried everything that has been suggested to no avail, you are left with no other alternative than to take a pill.

Like it or not, we have become a nation of pill-poppers. According to a 2004 report published by the U.S. Department of Health and Human Services, Americans consumed a whopping *45 percent* of the world's pharmaceuticals in the preceding year. That's a lot of pills and potions.

Why so many drugs? The faster-paced life becomes, the less we take care of ourselves, and the more day we steal from our night. You now understand all the negative health effects that sleep debt introduces into our lives. Compound that with all the emotional effects that living life at a breakneck pace can bring (anxiety, depression, panic attacks, and so on), and you begin to understand the need for so many pills.

It is natural to choose the path of least resistance. Why make life changes if you can get what you need from a pill? The problem with most medications is that they come with a dark side along with the temporary fix they provide. (Hence the long list of precautions and side effects in tiny letters that accompany every box, bottle, or drugstore bag.) Before taking any medication, and even before beginning a natural supplement, you should try to find out as much as you can about the product you intend to take. Only then will you be prepared to make a properly informed decision.

The History of the Sleeping Pill

The predicament of having trouble falling asleep or staying asleep probably dates back to post–Garden of Eden times. (I imagine Adam and Eve had a lot on their minds after being banished from the only garden they had ever known.) Sleeping pills have a much shorter history. The first to be produced and prescribed came from a family of drugs called *barbiturates*. (The same drugs that rock stars like Elvis Presley overdosed on.) Barbiturates were introduced in the early 1900s and remained the sleeping pills available until the late 1950s. They are powerful sedatives—so powerful that people still feel the effects the next morning. And as was the case with Elvis, a person can easily, and often unknowingly, take too much and wind up sedating themselves into a permanent nap.

Because inadvertent overdosing on barbiturates was happening with greater frequency, another group of sedating medications for the sleep-deprived population was introduced to the market in the late 1950s and early 1960s. *Benzodiazepines* are more commonly recognized by their brand names: Valium, Xanax, Halcion, and Librium. These had fewer serious side effects and potential hazards. Like barbiturates they are a central-nervous-system depressant—which is a fancy way to describe a sedative. This class of medications is still prescribed today to counteract short-term sleep problems, caused by such things as emotional trauma or physical pain. The downside is that they, like barbiturates, are highly addictive.

FALLING OVER WITH SLEEPING PILLS

The fact that sleeping pills work to make you sleepy is a good thing—as long as you are in bed, that is. But what if you have to get up early the next morning, or you awaken at midnight to use the bathroom? Well, here is where the trouble begins.

In 2004 the *British Medical Journal* published a study that looked at the effects of sedative-type sleeping pills on people 60 years and older. (It included a series of studies performed between 1966 and 2003.) Surprisingly, researchers discovered that for every one person who reported getting a better night's sleep while using sleeping pills, *two* seniors reported injuries from a trip, slip, or fall, or from an automobile accident while they were under the influence of sleeping pills.[1]

Just over two decades ago, the sleeping pill industry took a turn away from benzodiazepines and toward *sedative-hypnotic drugs*. According to Dr. Michael Nelson of Wingate University's College of Pharmacology, *sedative* refers to a substance that moderates activity and excitement while inducing a calming effect, while *hypnotic* refers to a substance that causes drowsiness and facilitates the onset and maintenance of natural sleep.[2]

In 1988, Ambien, the first of the new sedative-hypnotic sleeping aids, was introduced in Europe. Five years later it made its debut in the United States. Since its introduction here, Ambien has become the most frequently prescribed sleep medication in the U.S. Other hypnotic drug introductions soon followed—Lunesta, Sonata... with more to come, no doubt.

Knock Yourself Out

From the list above you can see that today there are a good number of relatively safe and effective nonbarbiturate, nonbenzodiazepine sleep medications that can help you to fall asleep faster or stay asleep longer. Yet each one comes with its own set of baggage. Let's run those bags through a "security checkpoint" so you can be fully informed of all they are packing before you allow them to board your body.

Ambien (four-hour formula) and Ambien CR (extended release)
Generic: Zolpidem

As I mentioned earlier, Ambien was introduced to the U.S. market in 1993. By the year 2005 a stunning 26.6 million prescriptions were written for it in that year alone.[3] With so many people taking this medication, some odd reports began to surface. Sleepwalking, sleep cooking, sleep eating, sleep sex…and most frightening, sleep *driving*.[4]

This last-listed oddity led Laura Liddicoat, a toxicologist from the state of Wisconsin, to present a paper at the American Academy of Forensic Sciences in February of 2006 entitled "Ambien—Drives Like a Dream?" Liddicoat was troubled by the increasing frequency that drivers, under the influence of remarkably high doses of Ambien, were crashing their cars with absolutely no memory of the incidents. It was discovered that the impaired drivers had exceeded the safe drug dose, had failed to put in the time needed to adequately sleep it off, or both. Now that's scary, wouldn't you agree?

The moral of this story is that you must first understand the working parameters of the medication you are on. For instance, the sleepy effects of Ambien, the four-hour sleep-*inducing* formula, will wear off after about four hours. On the other hand, Ambien CR, which is an extended-release medication, will be active in your body for a much longer time—upward of eight to ten hours.

Secondly, you cannot ignore your doctor's orders regarding the prescribed dosage. If you have become tolerant and are no longer experiencing the same sleep benefits you were, don't take it upon yourself to increase your dose. Put a call in to your physician and let them use their medical training to guide you. Don't go it alone—you may end up driving to Albuquerque in the middle of the night (or somewhere else if you already live in Albuquerque).

Finally, you must be aware of the potential for drug addiction. The original, short-acting Ambien is much more addictive by nature than the extended-release variety. For this reason, the latter can be used over a longer period of time without much risk of addiction.

Sonata
Generic: Zaleplon

After six years of being an only child in the prescription sleep-aid market, Ambien was joined in 1999 by another nonbenzodiazepine sibling—Sonata. Similar to the original Ambien (the non-CR variety), Sonata is a fast-acting medication capable of assisting a person in falling asleep. However, because it did not improve upon Ambien's mode of operation, it still lacked the staying power to assist in sleep maintenance beyond the first four hours.

RISKY BUSINESS

There are some things that rank worse than not sleeping well. Physical harm to you or your unborn baby could be an extremely unwanted outcome of taking prescription sleep medication. Sleeping pills should be avoided if you[5]

- have a history of depression, mental illness, or suicidal thoughts

- have a history of drug or alcohol abuse or addiction

- have liver or kidney disease

- are pregnant, are planning on getting pregnant, or are breastfeeding

- have sleep apnea

Some risks are not worth taking. "Better sleepy than sorry" is best for those of you who find yourself in one of the five categories above.

Lunesta
Generic: Eszopiclone

In 2005, the long-awaited new-generation sleeping pill, Lunesta, hit the market. This drug showed great promise in that it aided both in sleep initiation and sleep maintenance. It came complete with its own direct-to-consumer marketing plan. (You may associate this medication with a green butterfly that flutters about the bedroom.) This slick ad campaign had tired patients rushing to their physicians' offices asking for the "butterfly medication."

But all was not butterflies and rainbows for those taking Lunesta. Similar to its forerunner Ambien, it was found to reduce one's fear of risky behaviors, such as driving too fast, and its usage occasionally led to some of the bizarre sleep behaviors we spoke of earlier.[6]

Lunesta is a fast-acting sleep aid, as its two sedative-hypnotic predecessors are, so make sure you don't take it until you are ready to hop into bed. And because it has the added bonus of being long-acting, be sure you have set aside enough time to sleep it off as well.

Rozerem
Generic: Ramelteon

In July of 2005 a fourth sleep-aiding drug was approved for use in the U.S.—Rozerem. Like Lunesta, Rozerem is fast-acting and long-lasting. So if you do begin using this product, remember to take it immediately before bedtime and to remain in bed for the next eight hours or so.

Unfortunately, this drug is plagued with the same adverse side effects as the others. Here is a warning taken directly from the Rozerem website: "If you experience sleepwalking, driving, eating, or other behaviors *while not fully awake, without remembering the event*, contact your doctor immediately." (I've always wondered, if you don't remember those events having happened, how would you know to call your doctor the next morning?)

Cautions for Sleeping Pill Users

Your own prescription. Because of their addictive nature, sleeping pills are on the list of controlled substances here in the U.S. This means you must have a prescription for them in your own name. You should never, under any circumstances, take pills that have been prescribed for another person. Your doctor needs to examine *you* and take a thorough history to ensure your safety with any prescription medication.

Drowsiness and dullness. Sleeping pills should not be taken unless you are ready to dedicate the next seven to eight hours to sleep. They should never be used to enhance daytime napping, nor should some varieties be taken in the wee hours of the night when you have only a few hours left to sleep. And because all sleep medications dull your brain and render you less aware of your actions, don't take your evening dose until after you have finished all your evening activities (most importantly, driving). Not heeding this warning will certainly place you at greater risk for injury.

Alcohol use. When it comes to sleeping pills and alcohol use, one plus one equals four! Alcohol is a sedative on its own. The two used together can become a dangerous, and often a deadly mix. And remember, drinking alcohol within three hours of bedtime will work against your chances of getting a restful night's sleep, anyway.

Discontinuing use. Most physicians will tell their patients that prescription-based sleeping pills are to be used only for the short term—say for one to two weeks or so—because of both their addictive nature and because you can easily build up a tolerance to them. When you become tolerant of the dose you've been prescribed, it will no longer work effectively for you. When you're ready to stop taking your prescribed sleeping pills, follow your doctor's instructions or the directions on the label. Some medications must be discontinued gradually to avoid unwanted side effects.

Self-monitoring. Finally, be aware of how you feel the day *after* you've taken your prescribed medication. If you continue to feel sleepy after waking from a full night's sleep, or if you experience dizziness or a general light-headed feeling during the following day, inform your doctor right away. That particular medication may not be the right fit for you, or it might be that the dosage you've been prescribed is simply too high.

Over-the-Counter Sleep Aids

Most everyone who has struggled to sleep well has dabbled in the offerings of their drugstore's sleep-aids aisle. And who can be blamed? The television commercials are so convincing! For some people, this is all the help they ever need in their pursuit of a better night's sleep. I recall taking one of these nonprescription medicines one time following a couple frustrating nights of insomnia. I must say that although I did sleep, I did not feel well-rested and refreshed when I woke. Instead I felt rather groggy, like my head was full of cement—and this feeling lasted for at least the next two hours.

The point I am trying to make is that due to the intended drowsy effects of these sleeping aids, don't drive or attempt other activities that require alertness while under their influence. Some of the over-the-counter (nonprescription) medicines available today are listed below.

Sominex, Benadryl, Tylenol PM, Nytol

These medications all have one thing in common—their active ingredient is *diphenhydramine*. (Don't worry—you will not be asked to spell or pronounce that word.) Their side effects may include one or more of the following:[7]

- dry mouth
- dizziness
- prolonged drowsiness lasting into the next day
- headache
- loss of appetite
- gastrointestinal upset

All medications, whether they are prescription or nonprescription strength, must be filtered from our bodies by our livers and kidneys. Keep this in mind, as prolonged use of almost any medicine can have a deleterious effect on these organs. You'd do best not to take these meds if you are[8]

- pregnant
- breastfeeding

…or have a history of

- enlarged prostate
- glaucoma
- heart problems

NyQuil, Unisom

These medications have a different active ingredient, *doxylamine*, which may cause prolonged drowsiness, thus putting you at risk for accident or injury the following day. Again, do yourself a huge favor and do not take this group of meds if you are[9]

- pregnant
- breastfeeding

…or have a history of:

- asthma
- bronchitis
- enlarged prostate
- glaucoma
- peptic ulcer

IS TURKEY TRULY A SLEEP SUPPLEMENT?

Everyone seems to get sleepy after eating their annual Thanksgiving meal. So researchers set out to see if the turkey had anything to do with it. They found that this meat does indeed contain the chemical *tryptophan*, which is one of the two compounds necessary to produce the hormone melatonin. Aha!

Well, not so fast. Turkey doesn't contain much more tryptophan than chicken, fish, or a number of other foods we frequently eat. In fact, many of our daily diets contain foods much higher in tryptophan than turkey. So why all the Thanksgiving Day fatigue? Likely because we have stuffed ourselves as full as the bird on our tables. And if you have read either one of my books *Overcoming Overeating* or *Diabetes: Are You at Risk?*, you know that when your body digests a mother lode of food, your sugar levels spike. To protect you against a fainting episode (and other organ trauma) from such a high blood sugar level, your pancreas releases insulin, which rapidly counters the sharp rise in sugar. In doing so it overshoots and lowers your blood sugar past the point of normal—making you very, very *s-l-e-e-p-y*...

Natural Sleep Supplements

Some people find more comfort in taking something that is natural, rather than something man has produced in a laboratory. Unfortunately, the downside of this is that rigorous safety testing is done only on prescription and over-the-counter medications. Years of clinical trials precede the release of any new medication to the mass marketplace. Natural medicines and nutritional supplements do not undergo this process. And while they are regulated by the Food and Drug Administration (FDA), they do not undergo the same scrutiny by the FDA that prescription drugs do. In fact, it is the dietary supplement manufacturers who must tell the FDA that their products are safe and their label information is truthful.[10] The

FDA gets involved only after it receives consumer complaints about a product already on the market.

All this means you may not know what the long-term (or even short-term) effects of taking a supplement might be. Buyer, just beware.

Melatonin

We first mentioned melatonin back in chapter 2. It is one of the body's hormones; it assists in regulating our wake-sleep cycle. It is produced in a small part of the brain called the *pineal gland*. This gland, sometimes referred to as the third eye, is light-sensitive. The more light you are exposed to, the less melatonin you will make. As your Designer would have it, your body's peak production of melatonin is highest just before bedtime. The level of melatonin production does wane as we age, which may be one of the reasons older persons have difficulty sleeping.

It makes perfect sense that if melatonin is what prepares our body for sleep, than we would do well to give the body a dose of its own medicine. But here is where it gets a little tricky. Because we often lean toward "natural is better," a natural form of melatonin, harvested from the pineal glands of animals, can be found on the market today. Don't use it! Natural melatonin may pose a risk to humans because it can be contaminated with animal viruses. Synthetic melatonin is the way to go here because it is free from biological contaminants.[11]

So the real question is, Does melatonin work? I wish I had a really good answer to that really good question. Because melatonin has not been run through the extreme rigors of research testing that are routine for prescription and over-the-counter meds, the scientific jury is divided. The best we can do is to look to a watchdog group, the Natural Medicines Comprehensive Database, which rates the effectiveness of supplements and natural medicines based on the available scientific evidence. Once existing research studies have been reviewed, this group ranks their findings according to the following scale:

1. effective

2. likely effective

3. possibly effective

4. possibly ineffective

5. likely ineffective

6. ineffective

7. insufficient evidence to rate

According to this group, melatonin has been listed as "possibly effective" for jet lag and trouble sleeping (insomnia). The typical dose ranges from 0.3 to 5 milligrams per night. Follow the product instructions or ask your physician to determine what your dose should be.

Like anything you add to your body, you must be aware of the potential side effects of melatonin:

- daytime sleepiness
- dizziness
- headaches
- abdominal discomfort
- confusion
- sleepwalking
- nightmares

Furthermore, you may want to consult your doctor before using melatonin if you are pregnant or planning to become pregnant, or if you have any of these conditions:

- immune system disorder
- diabetes
- liver disease
- kidney disease

- history of stroke
- depression

As it does with other sleep aids, alcohol can exaggerate the effect of melatonin. Remember, too, that the next day you may find you are not entirely alert—so be sure to use extra precautions until you know how taking this supplement will affect you. By the way, melatonin is not recommended for people under 20. The National Institute of Health (NIH) has deemed it possibly unsafe because of its effects on other hormones, which might interfere with development during adolescence.[12]

Finally, be aware that melatonin may interact with various medications, including[13]

- blood-thinning medications (anticoagulants)
- immune system suppressants
- diabetes medications
- birth control pills

Valerian

If you frequent vitamin stores you may have come across the sleep-aid supplement valerian. Though not as popular as melatonin, valerian has been used for centuries as a natural sleep aid. Even Hippocrates recorded its sleep-inducing properties.

Valerian is a made from the roots of a flowering plant, which makes it more welcome to those seeking natural remedies. However, some of its baggage includes headache, excitability or uneasiness, and heart disturbances (such as racing). Once again, as with melatonin, the Natural Medicines Comprehensive Database has ranked it as being "possibly effective" for treating insomnia.[14]

Unlike melatonin, researchers have not been able to identify which chemical component of valerian is responsible for its sleepy effect. This has made it impossible to study its long-term effects or potential health hazards. So use the same precautions as you would with melatonin—don't use with alcohol, while pregnant, while breastfeeding, or while pursuing pregnancy.

With all the baggage these pills are packing, isn't it amazing that we are popping them at such a high rate? As I said at the outset of this chapter, my first recommendation is that you try everything else first—environment improvements, dietary changes, schedule revisions—everything, before you begin to alter your body's chemistry with medications. We still aren't sure what we don't know—but should—about these man-made sleep aids. So CAUTION: Pill-pop at your own risk.

A Final Good Night from Lisa

I don't know about you, but I've come a long ways from my earlier days, when I yawned over writing a book about sleep. How simply fascinating—and yet how wonderful complex—sleep is! My present understanding of its intricate architecture and its benefits has me thanking the Lord each night, as I lay my head down, for His gift. And each morning when I rise rested I am once again grateful for all the marvelous processes that have gone on in my body while I was unaware. Refreshed, renewed, and ready to begin the next day—a true miracle!

My newfound passion for the necessity of sound sleep—sound in both quality and quantity—has prompted me to begin speaking to groups on the subject. This is something I never imagined an orthopedic physical therapist would find herself doing! These presentations are among my audiences' favorites. And for good reason. Most of us, including me, have been ill-informed about our crucial need for 7 to 8 hours of sleep per night. Instead we have come to view it as merely a recommendation, one that carries no risk or impact if unheeded.

This book has been packed with research, respect, and concern for you, my reader. Your battle to win back the night will likely be victorious if you follow the advice I've laid out among its pages. My hope for you is that you will be able to rise up out of sleep debt, live life well-rested, and thus be empowered to age well, live long, and serve strong!

Good night, my new friend. I hope to hear great reports from a more well-slept you!

Lisa

Waking the Dead

10 Tips for Tired Teens

I have two teenagers at home who, during the school year, are rarely well rested. In order to catch their school bus in the morning, they must be up by 6:15 a.m. Watching them stand at the bus stop during the cold, winter months in the pitch dark, I wonder, Whose idea was this awful start time anyway? Surely school administrators and teachers must realize that high-schoolers need more sleep than they do.

While we adults need seven to eight hours to stay out of sleep debt, experts tell us that our teenagers need *9.25 hours* of sleep each night to meet the demands of their growing bodies![1] Given the school district's bus schedule, my teens would have to be asleep by 9:00 each night in order for them to be adequately rested. The likelihood of that occurring is slim to none—even though their mother is writing a book on sleep.

Trying to Do It All

The sad truth is, many of today's teens have been running on the hamster wheel ever since they were toddlers. And who put them there? Likely their parents. Moms and dads, thinking they are blessing their children, have loaded up their kids' schedules to the point where they are forced to scurry through their days at breakneck pace. On the other hand, there are some kids who come out of the womb wanting to experience it all—at the same time. And unfortunately, their parents make the mistake of allowing them to do just that: ballet, travel, soccer, karate, piano lessons, ice skating…all jammed into those precious nonschool hours. No one wins when life is lived at a frantic pace…no matter how many trophies are handed out.

By the time middle school rolls around, in addition to the smorgasbord of extracurricular activities, the students who show academic promise are fast-tracked (by their well-meaning teachers) into an aggressive learning stream that leads to a high-school schedule containing more college classes than high school ones. As the day draws to a close for these overextended teens, there is always more homework to be done, Facebook to check, bathing, and…*Okay, quick now—get to sleep, because tomorrow's another big day!*

The teens of this generation are burning the midnight oil in their struggle to fit it all in. When your day has no downtime, don't you find you can easily become overwhelmed and cranky? Yet we wonder why some of our teens sport bad grades, a poor attitude, and zombie-like behavior, which hangs over them like a gloomy cloud during what should be their brightest years. But can we really expect a different outcome with their demanding lifestyles?

And then there are those pockets of teens who are not overloaded by academic or extracurricular responsibilities, but have bought in hook, line, and sinker to the media blitz that is available to them 24-7. These kids lack the maturity to put boundaries up against the onslaught of external stimulation. No wonder they can't settle down. No wonder they can't avoid accumulating a huge load of sleep debt.

Side Effects of Teen Sleep Debt

Not only does lack of sleep make for a tired teen, but it also adds some very unwanted side effects. In one experiment, teenagers who slept less than six hours each night raised their susceptibility to the common cold virus by 50 percent.[2] This should not come as a surprise since we earlier discussed how the immune system is hamstrung without adequate sleep.

GET THOSE GRADES UP!

In 2002 a research study presented by Mary Carskadon of Cambridge University found that lack of sleep has a negative effect on teens' academic standing. (Is this surprising?) Reinforcing that point, Ms. Carskadon's study demonstrated that by sleeping just 17 to 33 minutes more per night, students were able to increase their school performance by an entire letter grade![3]

Another unwelcome side effect of sleep debt for teenagers is weight gain. Statistically one in every three children under 20 is overweight or obese. By the time they reach adulthood that number jumps to two out of three. Research has confirmed the relationship between sleep and weight by noting that any teenager who gets an average of less than six hours of sleep is 23 percent more likely to be obese.[4] So advise your teen to quit chasing after the latest fad diet and just go to bed earlier.

There is also a significant correlation between underslept teens and depression and suicidal thoughts. Researchers at Columbia University Medical Center found that students who went to bed after midnight were 24 percent more likely to report being depressed and 20 percent more likely to have suicidal thoughts when compared to teens whose bedtimes were set at 10:00 p.m. And even more frightening was that those teenagers who got five hours or less of sleep per night were *71 percent* more likely to report being depressed and *40 percent* more likely to think of suicide.[5]

Finally—and possibly the most dangerous to society at large—is the fact that teenage drivers—of whom 80 percent suffer from significant sleep debt—are statistically responsible for 50 percent of all automobile accidents.[6] Do you think there might be a correlation?

As I admitted at the start of this section, my teens do not get their full nine and a quarter hours of sleep most nights during the school year. That said, it seems (from what they say) that their sleep credit reports are stellar compared with those of their peers. My son manages to get about eight and a quarter hours of sleep on a school night and my daughter—who has a much heavier homework load—gets about seven.

From time to time I nudge them about getting more sleep. In response, both of them have told me that their friends frequently stay up till 1 or 2 a.m. to complete their homework assignments. When I ask for details about why their peers rack up such major sleep debt, I found out that many of the issues below were to blame. So with the intention of rescuing your teenagers from the plight of sleep debt—something that could plague them for the rest of their lives—we'll address these sleep depriving factors one by one.

1. Disconnect the media. Computer—shut it down. Laptop—close it. Television—turn it off. Movie—end it. Games—sign off. If your teen doesn't halt the continuous barrage of media streaming his way, there will be little chance he will successfully and rapidly switch from a highly roused state to restful slumber. My suggestion is to quit the use of all these visually stimulating devices *one hour* before bedtime. The human brain needs transition time.

2. Read before bed. Pre-bedtime pleasure reading (not a tedious English assignment) is a great way to disengage a teenager's brain from the day's activities. Just make sure the book isn't too compelling. They may be tempted to stay up late because each chapter ends in a cliff-hanger!

3. Silence the phone. The sleep of many teenagers is interrupted throughout the night simply because they don't silence their mobile phones. Text messages and phone calls sent in the wee hours of the morning rouse these media-plagued kids with strings of beeps and vibrations. And this generation feels compelled to answer every "poke," regardless of the time it occurs. Seriously, if your teen cannot disengage from their handheld device, maybe you need to babysit it for them while they sleep.

4. Dim the lights. Bright lights suppress melatonin production and confuse the body's built-in sleep timer. Teenagers already have a slightly skewed biological clock (which makes them stay up later and want to sleep in), so sitting in a brightly lit room or staring at a backlit computer screen before bedtime really works against production of their "sleepy hormone." Ease your teen into the night by dimming the lights around your home and in his room two hours before bedtime. Also, make sure they turn their face away from brightly lit screens (computer, iPad, TV, and so on) one hour prior to bedtime.

5. Cool down. Teenagers, with all their energy and enhanced hormone production, are often warmer than adults. Make sure their environment allows for the natural cooling of their bodies that is critical to initiating sleep. To ensure this, you may need to install a fan or an air conditioner in their bedroom.

6. Have a planned sleep schedule. Work with your teen to structure their day—work, extracurricular activities, and downtime—so they can get to bed at a reasonable time. Don't allow them to drastically alter their sleeping schedules during the weekend. This will only complicate matters during the week, when their biological clock must answer to their alarm clock.

7. Pack up the homework. If your teen claims they must stay up late to complete homework every night, then it's time to sit down with them and analyze their day. If there are too many other commitments, then decide which must be let go. If it seems to you that they are spending their homework time interacting on the computer or watching TV, then simply do not allow any media time until all their required work is complete. Your teen (and mine) knows how to work the situation to their advantage—if they tell us they are up late because of schoolwork, then what parent is going to make them go to bed? But if they were to finish their homework earlier in the day and then tell you they want to stay up to midnight watching their favorite DVR'd TV shows—any parent would pull the plug!

8. Quit the caffeine. Teenagers today are indulging in caffeinated drinks at an alarming rate—from lattes at Starbucks to Red Bulls and other "power drinks." It takes *six hours* for half of the caffeine your teen has consumed to be flushed from the body. Just as with adults, I recommend that no caffeine accompany dinner, and certainly do not allow them a big bowl of caffeine-containing chocolate or coffee-flavored ice cream for dessert.

9. Say no to nicotine. If your teenager has picked up the "cancer stick" habit, help him or her to understand that their body will have difficulty falling asleep with that stimulant racing through their bloodstream. Second, because of the addictive nature of nicotine, their body will wake up in the middle of the night in a state of withdrawal—whether or not they get out of bed to do something about that craving.

10. No late-night exercise. As mentioned earlier, the body must cool down as part of the preparation for sleep. If your teen is at a late-night hockey game or dance class, their bodies will be warm and toasty for an extended period of time afterward. This will work against the onset of sleep, even though they have played or practiced themselves into exhaustion. Your best bet is to wrap up all physical activities by 7:00 in the evening if your goal is a 10:00 p.m. lights-out.

Early on, my husband and I established a family rule that each child could participate in only two activities during the week. This was prompted by our desire to provide our kids with ample free time to create, recreate, and relate to other people in a noncontrolled setting. I also helped them manage their media time and schoolwork as they grew up so they had enough time to participate in everything that was important—including sleep.

As they have grown (they're now 15 and 17), my husband and I have cautiously allowed them to take on more responsibility and activity. Do I still micromanage their schedules? No. They have been trained so they can make time-healthy decisions on their own. And that was our goal all along. In just a short time Casey and Adam will leave the Morrone home for college, and I am confident they will be able to lead a balanced life that enables them to thrive, not just survive.

It is up to you, the parent of a sleep-challenged teen, to do everything you can in order to "train up your child in the way he should go, and when he is old, he will not depart from it" (Proverbs 22:6). A well-slept life is a productive life; a productive life is a blessed one.

Many blessings to you and your family
as you wisely seek to avoid sleep debt
and make good use of God's wonderful gift of sleep.
Lisa

Notes

Chapter 1–So Tired of Being Tired

1. eHealthMD, "What Is Insomnia?" www.ehealthmd.com/library/insomnia/ins_wha tis.html, accessed 2010 Oct 25.

2. A.N. Vgontzas, D. Liao, S. Pejovic, et al., "Insomnia with short sleep duration and mortality: the Penn State Cohort," *Sleep*, 2010; 33(9): 1159-64.

3. National Heart, Lung and Blood Institute, "What Causes Insomnia?" www.nhlbi.nih .gov/health/dci/Diseases/inso/inso_causes.html, accessed 2010 Oct 25.

Chapter 2–Eight Hours You Don't Want to Miss

1. Michael V. Vitiello and Bruce Nolan, "Sleep in America Poll," National Sleep Foundation, March 2, 2009.

2. Max Hirshkowitz and Patricia Smith, *Sleep Disorders for Dummies* (New York: Wiley Publishing, 2004), 70.

3. National Institute of General Medical Science (Division of the NIH), "Circadian Rhythms—Keeping Time," www.nigms.nih.gov/publications/factsheet_circadian rhythms.htm, accessed 2010 Oct 27.

4. Lawrence Epstein and Steve Mardon, *The Harvard Medical School's Guide to a Good Night's Sleep* (New York: McGraw-Hill, 2007), 18.

5. Manuel Schabus et al., "Sleep Spindles and Declarative Memory Consolidation," *Sleep*, 2004, 27(8): 1479-1485.

6. Suely Roizenblatt et al., "Alpha sleep characteristics in fibromyalgia," *Arthritis & Rheumatism*, 44: 222–230.

7. National Institute of Neurological Disorders and Strokes (Division of the NIH), www .ninds.nih.gov/disorders/brain_basics/understanding_sleep.htm, accessed 2010 Oct 27.

8. National Institute of Neurological Disorders and Stroke, "Brain Basics," accessed 2010 Nov 23.

9. National Institute of Neurological Disorders and Stroke.

Chapter 3—No Snooze? You Lose

1. Jane E. Ferrie et al., *Sleep,* 2007 December 1; 30(12): 1659–1666.

2. Institute for Natural Resources (INR), Seminar: "Brain Aging After 30," 2007.

3. J.P. Nilsson et al., "Less effective executive function after one night's sleep deprivation," *Journal of Sleep Research,* 2005 Mar; 14(1):1-6.

4. Paul E. Bendheim, *The Brain Training Revolution* (Naperville, IL: Source Books, 2009), 256-257.

5. Daniel Amen, *Making a Good Brain Great* (New York: Crown Publishing Group, 2005), 86.

6. M. Irwin, J. McClintick, C. Costlow, et al., "Partial night sleep deprivation reduces natural killer and cellular immune responses in humans," *FASEB Journal,* 1996; 10(5): 643-653.

7. Sanjay R. Patel and Frank B. Hu, "Short Sleep Duration and Weight Gain: A Systematic Review," *Obesity,* 2008; 16(3): 643-653.

8. Medline Plus, National Institute of Mental Health, "Depression," www.nlm.nih.gov/ medlineplus/depression.html, accessed 2010 Nov 23.

9. John Berman and Enjoli Francis, "AAA Says 2-of-5 Drivers Admit Nodding Off at the Wheel," ABC News, http://abcnews.go.com/WN/driving-sleepy-common-deadly- thought-aaa-research-finds/story?id=12088552, accessed 2010 Nov 8.

10. Deborah Kotz, "Driving Drowsy as Bad as Driving Drunk," *US News and World Report,* http://health.usnews.com/health-news/family-health/sleep/articles/2010/11/08/driv ing-drowsy-as-bad-as-driving-drunk.html, accessed 2010 Nov 23.

11. Berman and Francis.

12. Murray Johns, "The Epworth Sleepiness Scale," Stanford University website, www .stanford.edu/~dement/epworth.html, accessed 2010 Nov 24.

Chapter 4—Getting Ready for a Good Night's Sleep

1. James Maas and Rebecca Robbins, *Sleep for Success* (Bloomington, IN: AuthorHouse, 2010), 84.

2. Lawrence Epstein and Steve Mardon, *The Harvard Medical School's Guide to a Good Night's Sleep* (New York: McGraw-Hill, 2007), 63.

3. Epstein and Mardon, 64.

4. Ryan Hurd, "What are sleep treatments for jet lag?" LiveStrong.com. www.livestrong .com/article/94190-sleep-treatments-jet-lag/, accessed 2010 Dec 15.

5. Hurd.

6. Epstein and Mardon, 56.

Chapter 5—"Oh No, I've Gotta Go!"

1. L. Yoffee, medically reviewed by Lindsey Marcellin, "Medications used to treat

hypertension," Everyday Health. www.everydayhealth.com/hypertension/treating/medications-used-to-treat-hypertension, accessed 2011 Jan 4.

2. Michael Bihari, "Can I Take Lipitor or Zocor with Grapefruit Juice?" About.com, December10,2008,http://drugs.about.com/od/faqsaboutyourdrugs/f/statins_grapefr.htm, accessed 2011 Jan 4.

3. Michael Safir, Clay Boyd, and Tony Pinson, *Overcoming Urinary Incontinence* (Omaha, NE: Addicus Books, 2008), 9.

4. Medline Plus, National Library of Medicine/National Institute of Health, "Enlarged Prostate," www.nlm.nih.gov/medlineplus/ency/article/000381.htm, accessed 2011 Jan 6.

5. eHealthMD.com, "Normal Prostate Growth During Life," www.ehealthmd.com/library/prostateenlargement/BPH_causes.html, accessed 2011 Jan 11.

6. The American Cancer Society, www.cancer.org, www.cancer.org/cancer/prostatecancer/detailedguide/prostate-cancer-key-statistics, accessed 2011 Jan 10.

7. Paul Lange and Christine Adamec, *Prostate Cancer for Dummies* (New York: Wiley Publishing, Inc., 2003), 26.

8. National Association for Continence, www.nafc.org, www.nafc.org/index.php?page=prolapse#5, accessed 2011 Jan 19.

Chapter 7–The Sleep Apnea Emergency

1. www.MayoClinic.com, www.mayoclinic.com/health/sleep-apnea/DS00148/ DSEC TION = symptoms, accessed 2011 Feb 24.

2. T.D. Bradley and J.S. Floras, "Obstructive sleep apnea and its cardiovascular consequences," *Lancet,* 2009; 373: 82-93.

3. Lawrence Epstein and Steve Mardon, *The Harvard Medical School's Guide to a Good Night's Sleep* (New York: McGraw-Hill, 2007), 130.

4. Siamak Nabili and Andrew Verneuil, MedicineNet.com, www.medicinenet.com/sleep_apnea/page6.htm#toch, accessed 2011 February 16.

5. Brandon Peters, "Definition of AHI," About.com, January 26, 2011, http://sleepdisorders.about.com/od/glossary/g/AHI.htm, accessed 2011 March 9.

6. S. Redline and P.V. Tishler, "The Genetics of Sleep Apnea," *Sleep Medicine Reviews,* 2000 Dec; 4(6): 583-602.

7. N.S. Marshall et al., "Sleep apnea as an independent risk factor for all-cause mortality: The Busselton Health Study," *Sleep,* 2008; 31: 1079-1085.

8. "Sleep-Disordered Breathing and Mortality: Eighteen-Year Follow-Up of the Wisconsin Sleep Cohort," *Sleep,* August 1, 2008.

9. "Heart Disease and Stroke Statistics—2006 Update: a report from the AHA statistics committee and stroke statistics subcommittee," *Circulation* 2006; 113: 85-181.

10. P.L. Smith, A.R. Gold, et al., "Weight Loss in Mildly to Moderately Obese Patients with OSA," *Annals of Internal Medicine* 1985; 103: 850-855.

Chapter 8–Restless Legs Syndrome

1. www.MayoClinic.com, "Restless Legs Syndrome: Treatment and Drugs," www.Mayo Clinic.com/health/restless-leg-syndrome/DS00191/ DSECTION =treatments-and-drugs, accessed 2011 Feb 2.

2. Mark Buchfuhrer, Wayne Hening, and Clete Kushida, *Restless Legs Syndrome* (St. Paul, MN: American Academy of Neurology Press, 2007), 6.

3. M. Bayard, T. Avonda, and J. Wadzinski, "Restless leg syndrome," *American Family Physician,* 2008 Jul 15; 78(2): 243.

4. National Institute of Neurological Disorders and Stroke, www.nainds.nih.gov, www.ninds.nih.gov/disorders/restless_legs/detail_restless_legs.htm, accessed 2011 Feb 1.

5. Clete Kushida, "Clinical presentation, diagnosis, and quality of life issues in restless legs syndrome," *American Journal of Medicine,* 2007 Jan; 120(1 Suppl 1): S4-S12.

6. www.MayoClinic.com.

7. www.MayoClinic.com.

8. National Institute of Neurological Disorders and Stroke.

9. www.MayoClinic.com.

10. National Institute of Neurological Disorders and Stroke.

11. Buchfuhrer et al., 106-107.

Chapter 9–Attack of the Busy Brain

1. Psalm 4:8.

2. 2 Corinthians 10:5.

3. Ephesians 4:26.

4. Ephesians 4:26.

Chapter 10–"Just Take a Pill…"

1. J. Glass et al., "Sedative hypnotics in older people with insomnia: meta-analysis of risks and benefits," *British Medical Journal,* November 2005; 331(7526): 1169.

2. M. Nelson, "Sedative-Hypnotic Drugs," Pharmacy 725: Principles of Drug Mechanisms, Wingate University School of Pharmacy, http://pharmacy.wingate.edufaculty/mnelson/PDF/Sedative_Hypnotics.pdf, accessed 2011 March 21.

3. "Popular Sleeping Pill Linked to 'Sleep Driving,' *New York Times* Reports," www.Fox News.com. Wednesday, March 08, 2006, www.foxnews.com/story/0,2933,187230,00.html, accessed 2011 March 22.

4. www.fda.gov, "Zolpidem" pdf download, 13 Sept 2008. www.fda.gov/downloads/Drugs/DrugSafety/ucm089833.pdf, accessed 2011 March 28; National Center for Biotechnology Information/National Library of Medicine/National Institutes of Health, PubMed Health, "Zolpidem," September 2008, www.ncbi.nlm.nih.gov/pubmed health/PMH0000928/, accessed 2011 March 28.

5. www.MayoClinic.com, "Insomnia/Prescription Sleeping Pills: What's Right for You?" www.MayoClinic.com/health/sleeping-pills/SL00010, accessed 2011 March 28.

6. www.lunesta.com, "Medication Guide" ©2010, www.lunesta.com/Lunesta-Patient-Medication-Guide.pdf?iid=body_medGuide, accessed 2011 March 28.

7. Maryanne Hochadel, *The AARP Guide to Pills* (New York: Sterling Publishing Company, 2007), 280.

8. Hochadel, 279.

9. www.nlm.nih.gov, MedlinePlus, "Doxylamine," www.nlm.nih.gov/medlineplus/druginfo/meds/a682537.html, accessed 2011 March 28.

10. www.fda.gov, The Food and Drug Administration, "Dietary Supplements," www.fda.gov/food/dietarysupplements/default.htm, accessed 2011 March 24.

11. Brent A. Bauer, "Sleep Aids," www.MayoClinic.com, www.mayoclinic.com/health/sleepaids/SL00016/NSECTIONGROUP=2, accessed 2011 March 23.

12. www.nlm.nih.gov, The National Library of Medicine, Medline Plus, "Melatonin," www.nlm.nih.gov/medlineplus/druginfo/natural/940.html, accessed 2011 March 24.

13. Brent A. Bauer, "Melatonin side effects: What are the risks?" www.MayoClinic.com, www.mayoclinic.com/health/sleepaids/SL00016/NSECTIONGROUP=2, accessed 2011 March 24.

14. www.nlm.nih.gov, The National Library of Medicine, Medline Plus, "Valerian," www.nlm.nih.gov/medlineplus/druginfo/natural/870.html, accessed 2011 March 24.

Bonus Section: Waking the Dead

1. James Maas and Rebecca Robbins, *Sleep for Success* (Bloomington, IN: AuthorHouse, 2010), 115.

2. Maas and Robbins, 112.

3. Mary A. Carskadon, *Adolescent Sleep Patterns: Biological, Social, and Psychological Influences* (Cambridge, UK: Cambridge University Press, 2002).

4. Maas and Robbins, 113.

5. James Gangwisch et al., "Earlier Parental Set Bedtimes as a Protective Factor Against Depression and Suicidal Ideation," *Sleep*, 2010 Jan 1; 33: 97-106.

6. Maas and Robbins, 114.

About the Author

Lisa Morrone graduated magna cum laude from the physical therapy program at the State University of New York at Stony Brook in 1989, receiving a Bachelor of Science degree in Physical Therapy. In addition to her college education, Lisa has taken over 30 continuing education courses in the area of orthopedic physical therapy. As a physical therapist, Lisa has been treating patients in the field of orthopedic rehabilitation for over two decades. In 1990 she accepted the position of adjunct professor at Touro College, Bay Shore, New York, which she still holds today.

At Touro College Lisa instructs in the Entry Level Doctorate Program in Physical Therapy. Each fall semester she teaches Musculoskeletal II (Spinal Orthopedics). Her past teaching credits include: Spinal Stabilization Training, Spinal Muscle Energy Techniques, Massage, Extremity Joint Mobilization (evaluation and treatment of the joints in the arms and legs), and Kinesiology (the study of bones, muscles, and joints and their roles in the human body).

Lisa's library of self-help books began with *Overcoming Back and Neck Pain*, published in February 2007, and with this latest addition numbers half a dozen books. Lisa is a graduate of both the speaker and the writer tracks of the She Speaks Conference (Proverbs 31 Ministries), where she was assessed at the highest level of proficiency. As a speaker, Lisa has taught in both secular (community and medical) and church-based settings. Additionally, she is a regular health contributor for the online magazine *Living Better at 50+* and has been a regular guest on Moody Radio's *This Is the Day*. Lisa makes her home on Long Island, New York, along with her husband, daughter, and son.

Restoring Your Temple™

Within Christian circles, one's physical body is often referred to as the temple of the Holy Spirit. The reason for this is found in 1 Corinthians 6:19, where the Bible says, "Do you not know that your body is a temple of the Holy Spirit, who is in you, whom you have received from God?" Temples are places where worship takes place. But what exactly is worship? To quote author Rick Warren,

> Worship is far more than praising, singing, and praying to God. Worship is a lifestyle of *enjoying* God, *loving* him and *giving* ourselves to be used for his purposes. When you use your life for God's glory, everything you do can become an act of worship.

Romans 12:1 further tells us to "offer your *bodies* as living sacrifices, holy and pleasing to God—this is your spiritual act of worship." God has plans for your body...physical plans. Your hands and feet are meant to be used as His hands and feet on this earth. So whether He calls you to raise children, teach Sunday school, or work with teenagers or the homeless, you need a physical body that is ready for action. Scripture says, "The harvest is plentiful, but the workers are few." Oftentimes this is because the workers are at a doctor's appointment, are going to physical therapy, or are simply so tired they can't get off the couch!

It is the intent of **Restoring Your Temple** to ready the Body of Christ to perform the work of Christ. The longer you live in good physical health, the greater your capacity to serve God will be, and the more you will be able to enjoy the abundant life He has promised to His children.

Visit Lisa's website, **www.LisaMorrone.com,** for free resources that include

- a BMI (body mass index) calculator
- a home exercise program for those suffering with jaw pain (TMD)
- downloadable headache tracking charts
- guidance on how to find a good physical therapist
- a source of "Lisa-tested," quality health-related products
- quick tips for back, neck, head, or jaw pain and blood-sugar regulation
- helpful articles on health-related issues
- photos of proper sleeping postures
- the complete library of Lisa's books, including *Overcoming Headaches and Migraines*

Also by Lisa Morrone, PT

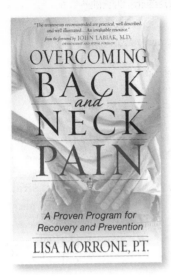

Overcoming Back and Neck Pain

A Proven Program for Recovery and Prevention

"The treatments Lisa recommends are practical, well described, and well illustrated...An invaluable resource."

FROM THE FOREWORD BY JOHN LABIAK, MD,
ORTHOPAEDIST AND SPINAL SURGEON

From 20 years of teaching and practicing physical therapy, Lisa Morrone gives you a way to say *no* to the treadmill of prescriptions, endless treatments, and a limited lifestyle. This straightforward, clinically proven approach offers the most effective exercises, guidelines, and lifestyle adjustments for back and neck problems, showing you how to...

- benefit from good posture and "core stability"
- strengthen and stretch key muscles
- shift to healthy movement patterns
- recover from pain caused by compressed or degenerated discs
- address "inside issues" that affect your body's healing capacity—nutrition, rest, and emotional/spiritual struggles

With Lisa's help, you can gain freedom from pain—and regain your freedom to enjoy work, friends, family, and a fulfilling life.

"This book takes a very practical approach to the key things patients really need to know."

KENT KEYSER, MS, PT, OCS, COMT, ATC, FFCFMT, FAAOMPT
PRACTICING AND TEACHING PHYSICAL THERAPIST

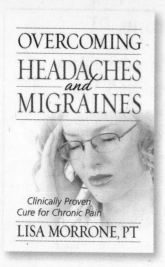

OVERCOMING
HEADACHES
and
MIGRAINES

*Clinically Proven
Cure for Chronic Pain*

LISA MORRONE, PT

Overcoming Headaches and Migraines

Clinically Proven Cure for Chronic Pain

"A gift to headache sufferers and those in the health professions who are committed to helping them."

—HOWARD MAKOFSKY, PT, DHSc, OCS HEAD PAIN EXPERT

If you're one of the millions who experience chronic or debilitating headaches and are looking for practical help and answers, physical therapist Lisa Morrone has them. Nearly 20 years of teaching, research, and hands-on treatment have given her a thorough, broad-based perspective on head pain.

As a headache or migraine sufferer, you don't have to resign yourself to being a pill-popping victim. Instead, you can achieve lasting changes by discovering how to...

- uncover the source of your head pain and avoid unnecessary medication
- eliminate pain originating from neck problems or muscle tension
- ward off migraines and cluster headaches by pinpointing and avoiding your "triggers"
- decide whether self-treatment, treatment by a practitioner, or a combination of both is best
- find a qualified hands-on practitioner
- get free from the emotions of anger and anxiety that can keep you trapped in head pain

This comprehensive resource combines effective habits, exercises, and lifestyle adjustments to help you end head-pain disability and get back a life you can enjoy and share.

"A complete and understandable guide for both the practitioner and the patient."

—WILLIAM ROBERT SPENCER, MD, FAAP; EAR, NOSE, AND THROAT SPECIALIST

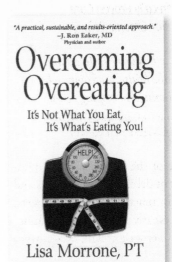

"A practical, sustainable, and results-oriented approach."
–J. Ron Eaker, MD
Physician and author

Overcoming Overeating

It's Not What You Eat,
It's What's Eating You!

Lisa Morrone, PT

Overcoming Overeating

It's Not What You Eat,
It's What's Eating You!

Health author Lisa Morrone bypasses diet plans and zeros in on *heart* plans—because food isn't typically the real problem. Here are tools to assess *yourself* (not just your food intake), followed by tested methods for breaking through the food trap from the inside out. You'll find ways to

- identify and address the underlying causes of your overeating
- avoid using food as a time-filler, mood elevator, or painkiller
- find freedom to achieve steady, solid results from any reputable weight-loss method
- *finally* keep the weight off, feel better about yourself, and improve your overall health

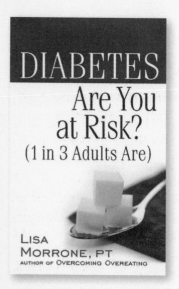

Diabetes

Are You at Risk? (1 in 3 Adults Are)

You could be one of the 60 million American adults with prediabetes. Why? Because most people with this condition *don't know they have it*. And an additional 7 million adults don't know they have full-blown diabetes!

Diabetes: Are You at Risk? will help you find out where *you* stand. Better yet, it will show you how to stop or even reverse the consequences of untreated blood-sugar problems. Health author Lisa Morrone gives you the tools to set a new course:

- a self-quiz to assess your current condition
- a concise understanding of how your body processes blood sugar
- a summary of the progressive problems caused by poorly regulated blood sugar
- step-by-step changes in eating habits that can preserve or restore your health
- easy ways to "get yourself moving" so your body can enjoy the diabetes-fighting benefits of physical activity

This can-do, action-oriented resource points the way toward a longer, healthier, more productive life—a life that will benefit you and those close to you.

More Harvest House Resources
to Help You Help Yourself

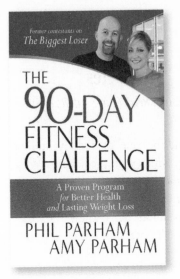

The 90-Day Fitness Challenge

A Proven Program for Better Health and Lasting Weight Loss

PHIL AND AMY PARHAM

You've tried the diet plans with little success. Now let Phil and Amy Parham, former contestants on NBC's *The Biggest Loser,* show you how to transform your life and live your dreams of being healthier, happier, and more fit. *The 90-Day Fitness Challenge* is a faith-based, informative, and motivational book that will

- take you step-by-step through a 90-day program for permanent weight loss
- provide you simple and practical healthy food and fitness plans
- point the way toward developing better eating habits and an active lifestyle
- incorporate Scripture and faith principles to encourage you to make God a part of your journey

The Parhams know from experience the obstacles to fitness that you face. Allow them to come alongside to inspire, motivate, and provide practical life skills on your 90-day journey toward better health and lasting weight loss.

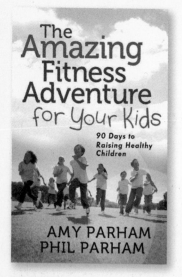

The Amazing Fitness Adventure for Your Kids

90 Days to Raising Healthy Children

PHIL AND AMY PARHAM

Childhood obesity is on the rise. Many kids—perhaps even your own—would rather play video games or watch TV than run around a playground or in their backyard. The damage to their health is alarming.

But there is hope. This inspirational and easy-to-follow guide is filled with tips from Phil and Amy Parham's own family journey and will show you

- creative ways to be physically active as a family
- simple ways to prepare nutritious meals and snacks
- fun and rewarding ways to make a healthy lifestyle a habit

The Amazing Fitness Adventure for Your Kids gives you not only the tools to raise fit kids but also a road map to the rewards that come from enjoying a healthy lifestyle together—stronger and healthier kids and a more closely knit family.

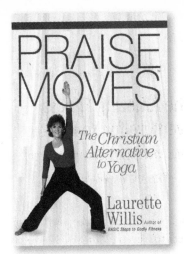

PraiseMoves™
The Christian Alternative to Yoga
LAURETTE WILLIS

Would you like to increase your flexibility, improve your circulation, and enhance your level of energy? Finally there's a program that offers proven stretching and flexibility exercises without troubling Eastern influences. Now you can fill your mind with the Word of God as you practice the postures on this DVD that will

- promote healing and overall physical health
- relieve stress and enhance relaxation
- glorify God with your spirit, soul, and body

Renew your mind...rejuvenate your body. Certified personal trainer Laurette Willis shows you a way to transform your workouts into worship with *PraiseMoves*™.

To learn more about other Harvest House books
or to read sample chapters, log on to our website:

www.harvesthousepublishers.com

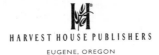

HARVEST HOUSE PUBLISHERS

EUGENE, OREGON